# Raw
# CAN CURE
# CANCER

## HIGHLIGHTS FROM
## A TRUE STORY

JANETTE MURRAY-WAKELIN

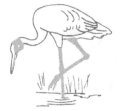

Published by Brolga Publishing Pty Ltd
ABN 46 063 962 443
PO Box 12544
A'Beckett St
Melbourne, VIC, 8006
Australia

email: markzocchi@brolgapublishing.com.au

All details can be found in National Library of Australia Cataloguing-in-Publication entry database
Author:          Murray-Wakelin, Janette.
Title:            Raw can cure cancer : 100% raw courage: a journey to optimum
                  health / Janette Murray-Wakelin. (edition 3)
ISBN:            9781922175779 (pbk.)

*In Memory of*
*my beloved parents*
*who showed me the true meaning of unconditional love*


*Dedicated to*
*my partner in life, my children and grandchildren*
*who show me the true meaning of happiness*


*Special Thanks*
*to all the kind, caring and compassionate people*
*who show me the true meaning of life*

# CONTENTS

# FOREWORD

I n 2001 I was diagnosed with highly aggressive carcinoma breast cancer. I was 52 years old, a mother of two and grandmother of one. I was told I had six months to live.

I was not willing to accept this prognosis, which prompted me to search for a way other than what was being offered to me by the conventional medical process. I discovered truths and lies about cancer. This led me to making conscious lifestyle choices that have changed my life forever.

Within six months I received a clean bill of health and as a result of my life changing experience, established a Raw Vegan Restaurant and Centre for Optimum Health where I offered Raw Conscious Lifestyle Programs based on the holistic approach of mind, body and spirit.

Ten years after my 'death sentence' I wrote 'Raw Can Cure CANCER – Highlights from aTrue Story'.

This story is the compilation of the highlights of events that really occurred and conversations that really took place. I have fictionalised my story by changing the names and adding excerpts from stories that other women shared, but I emphasise that **this story is all based on fact.**

Prevention is the key to optimum health and everyone has a choice about how well they want to live. The cure for cancer has become a big money making industry, but people who are diagnosed with cancer have a choice that many are unaware of. It is my hope that this story opens up the possibility of what we can achieve when we choose to live with WELLNESS.

While there are highs and lows to every story, it is the highlights of a story that remain as knowledge. I encourage you, my reader, to highlight passages throughout this book for easy reference to the questions and answers that may resonate for you. May every choice you make in life be born of a simple conscious thought.

To inspire and motivate conscious lifestyle choices, to promote kindness and compassion to all living beings and to raise environmental awareness for a sustainable future, as veteran raw vegan ultra endurance athletes, my partner and I are running around Australia, 15,500 kilometres, a marathon a day for 365 days, throughout 2013. **www.RawVeganPath.com**

— Janette Murray-Wakelin
2013

# FOREWORD BY DR. IAN GAWLER

Those of you with faint hearts, do not go here. *Raw Can Cure Cancer* is a book for people with intelligence and courage. In it, Janette Murray –Wakelin uses superb narrative to chronicle her recovery from advanced secondary breast cancer using a wide range of natural therapies. In the process, she draws into question and challenges many societal norms, but then, she is alive to do so.

Janette's voice is that of direct experience backed by thorough investigation. Her book warrants wide readership and could well save the lives of others.

The fact is that for many, the fear that rushes in to accompany a diagnosis of cancer often crushes their courage and over-rides their intelligence. As a consequence, they have difficulty thinking or acting for themselves.

*Raw Can Cure Cancer* demonstrates another possibility. Janette responded to her diagnosis in 2001 by questioning everything. Everything. She did this systematically, not necessarily without some strong initial emotions, but then she took the time to consult, research and reflect. Janette thought all her options through thoroughly, and then she made deliberate, conscious choices.

Next, Janette displayed her courage. Having accepted initial, localised surgery, but then having decided that in her mind the small possible benefits from additional medical treatment were outweighed by the risks of side-effects, Janette committed to "the road less travelled". She refused the recommended on-going medical treatment and opted for an all-natural approach.

Nervous? Some diagnosed with cancer say timidly "Who am I to question my doctors?" Others might say "I only want to do what the family is happy with. Don't want to rock the boat." Some authorities may well prefer these matters were not being presented and discussed.

However, Janette did dare to think and to act for herself. She stood strong in the face of medical criticism for her choices. She remained steadfast while friends and even family questioned her motives, her thinking, her conclusions. With courage she persevered, gathered a supportive team and prevailed. She recovered fully.

And then of course, in 2013, almost by way of celebration, certainly as a statement, she wrote herself into the record books by running around Australia with her husband, completing a full marathon every day for a year and one day – all on raw food.

*Raw Can Cure Cancer* is fascinating, challenging, informative, timely. Not for the faint hearted. But do have the courage, Use your intelligence. Read it. Give it those you are close to – a great book to read when you are well or when in need. Think about it. Discuss it. Make up your own mind.

May you live a long and happy life

— **Dr Ian Gawler OAM, BVSc, MCounsHS**
**Author of You Can Conquer Cancer**
**www.iangawler.com**
**Yarra Junction, May 2014**

# CHAPTER 1
## A PRECIOUS GIFT

Ariena wandered happily around the festival, pausing at the various booths to admire the artwork on display. Artists and photographers, painters and potters, wood turners and crafts people, musicians and performers, all with their brightly coloured banners and booths were intermingled with a variety of food stalls of all flavours. The spicy aroma of Indian fare, the sweet smell of sugary delights, the fresh scent of salads and sandwiches and freshly squeezed lemonade, and a sniff of salt in the air, all wafted on the breeze tantalising the tastebuds. Children chased each other through the park, ducking in and out of the booths and stalls, squealing with excitement and delight while parents and grandparents walked along discussing the arts and crafts that caught their attention, occasionally glancing towards their children and grandchildren, knowing they were safe to play freely within this community.

Ariena noticed her daughter Joy looking at a display of hand made tie-dyed scarves, while holding her baby son Kenny. Smiling at her mother and knowing there was no need to ask, Joy said, "Can you hold him while I go get some food for us?" Ariena's heart melted as the little boy, not quite one year old, reached out his chubby hands to her.

"Come to Nannie," Ariena said, "we'll go find the animals to talk to." She kissed his little button nose and he chuckled, wrapping his arms around her neck. The petting farm had goats and sheep, ducks and chickens, rabbits and guinea pigs, and an old grey donkey, all

1

busy eating the hay that had been scattered on the ground for them. Ariena walked into the pen and squatted down close to the animals so her grandson could see them.

"Reach out your hand and they may come to you, then you can gently stroke them. They like that," she told him. The goats came bounding over and tried to nibble his hand, making him giggle. The ducks waddled along, quacking their arrival noisily. The chickens pecked at the ground, absently clucking to each other, and while the rabbits hopped happily about, the guinea pigs ran wildly in all directions. Kenny clapped his hands together and laughed out loud. The old grey donkey wandered over and sniffed at him, its velvety muzzle tickling his neck. He reached out and tentatively stroked his fingers on the softness of the animal's nose, delighting in the warm touch. A large and woolly sheep walked up and rubbed against them, almost knocking them over. They both laughed as the sheep looked at them questioningly. Kenny closed his fingers around a handful of wool and pulled himself close enough to rub his face in the softness of it.

Ariena smiled and lay her cheek on the animal's back facing her grandson. He lifted his head and kissed her, then buried his face in the thick wool and kissed the sheep. The child's display of unconditional love gave Ariena a lump in her throat and she had to blink back the tears of love she felt for him. She sat him on her knee and picked up a tiny rabbit with floppy ears. Carefully she placed it on Kenny's lap. His face lit up with joy and he wrapped his arms around the fluffy bunny. The little furry nose stopped twitching and the rabbit closed its eyes. Kenny stroked its head and, lifting his finger to his mouth whispered, "Shhh," to his grandmother. Ariena's heart melted. As she looked down at Kenny's hand gently holding the little paw, her mind went back to almost a year before when he was only a few hours old. While he lay in a crib, his tiny fingers had held tightly onto her hand and Ariena recalled how she had whispered that she would always be there for him. She noticed how the little rabbit's whiskers twitched as it slept and remembered her grandson's eyelids fluttering as he had slept the exhausted sleep of a newborn. Now, his fingers slowly uncurled and his hand flopped onto his lap, the little rabbit did not move. Ariena looked at his sleeping face and that of the bundle of fur on his lap, and smiled. *Babies are such a precious gift*, she thought. She carefully placed the sleeping bunny on a thick pile of hay and lifted Kenny to her chest. He stirred and clutched onto her with his little hand, falling back into a deep contented sleep.

Holding her precious bundle close to her, she walked through the surrounding festive atmosphere towards the picnic area. A warm arm wrapped around her shoulder as her husband whispered, "We're all gathering for lunch, come and join us." He stepped forward offering to take the sleeping child. She smiled and shook her head. "Let's not disturb him," she said. "I'll hold him for a while, he'll be fine." Glen slipped his arm around her waist and they walked companionably together.

"Brings back memories, doesn't he?" he said, nodding towards their grandson.

"Yes, sure does," she agreed.

Sitting at the picnic table, sharing the meal with her family, Ariena continued to hold her sleeping bundle while she ate, sitting beside Glen who kept his arm around her and chatting with her own parents who had joined them for the day's outing. She felt very happy with her life and couldn't help thinking how blessed she was.

How could she know that in an instant, everything would change...

# CHAPTER 2
## LOVE

Ariena gently placed her sleeping grandson in his stroller.

"He's getting heavy," she said as she put him down.

"You could have put him down long ago," Joy commented, giving her mother a pat on the shoulder.

"I know," Ariena smiled. She stretched the kinks out of her back and rubbed her breast where Kenny had been holding on to her as he slept.

"He's got quite the grip for a little guy," she said with a grin. Then the smile left her face, replaced with a frown and a puzzled look.

"Mum, what's wrong?"

Ariena felt a wave of foreboding sweep over her.

"Mum, what is it?"

"Oh, it's probably nothing," Ariena said dismissively.

"What's probably nothing? Mum?"

Ariena looked at her daughter. "Well, I thought I felt a lump in my breast, but it's most likely just bruised from the tight grip your son had on me," she reasoned with a laugh.

"Whatever it is, you had better have it checked out." Joy turned to her father. "Dad, will you make sure she does?"

"Don't worry," he winked trying to make light of the situation. He put his arm around Ariena and gave her a squeeze.

"Trust me, I'll take care of her." As he kissed her affectionately on her head, he whispered in her ear, "Nothing a little bit of love wont take care of."

"Yes," Ariena replied with a knowing smile.

Ariena placed her hand on Glen's knee as he drove them home. He reached down and squeezed her hand and smiled at her briefly. Neither of them said anything. They were both thinking and hoping the same thing, *it's nothing, everything will be fine.* Her thoughts went back over the years she and Glen had spent together. How young they had been when they were married more than thirty years ago, and how much in love they had been then. She remembered the joy of their wedding day and how gentle he had been with her on their wedding night. *How naive I was*, she thought, remembering how unprepared she was for the moments of deep passion and pleasure she experienced for the first time as he made love to her. She chuckled to herself as she remembered writing to her mother the next day, telling her how surprised she was that making love could be so delightful! She remembered how, after their honeymoon they settled into married life easily, going back to work separately, but coming home to each other and the deep love they shared together. She remembered how, after they made love, she would be overcome with a mixture of joy and fear, a fear that she might lose him one day. He had asked her, *If you are so happy why are you crying?* She had voiced her fear to him then and he had reassured her, *I'm not going anywhere, I'll always be here to take care of you.* She thought of the pure happiness that birthing their two children had brought to her and how her love for her husband had deepened then. She thought about all the happy times they spent with the children, growing together, working and playing together. Her mind marvelled at how much love could be shared in a family and what a precious gift her children were. She recalled the moments of laughter and joy their little ways brought and she recalled the mixture of joy and concern as they grew. She remembered the moments of fear, dread, anxiety and eventually relief, when their little son Scott had endured hours of heart surgery, pain and healing. She remembered how, in his hardest moments, he tried to appear tough and gave her the 'thumbs up'. She remembered the moments of love and pride she felt for her little girl when Joy refused to leave her little brother's bedside.

"Not until he is feeling better," Joy had said in her best attempt at a grown-up voice. She thought how determined Joy had been to protect Scott and how the love her two children shared had never waned. She felt again the touch of Glen's hand on her shoulder as he had tried to comfort her, holding her close as they watched over their children. Memories came flooding back of the happiness and relief they had felt when all was well and how thankful they were for the caring expertise of the doctor who had done so much for their son. She smiled to herself as she remembered how Glen had been so relieved, he had enthusiastically pumped the surgeon's hand squeezing his fingers, before suddenly realising that that was probably not such a good idea!

*

As she continued to gaze out the window, she remembered with melancholy the troubled times they had had as a couple, when again the fear of losing him came so close to reality. *How many tears of anguish did I cry? How deep was my despair. How unworthy I thought I was. How unattractive I thought I must have become. How low my self-esteem stooped that I felt the need to prove myself and retaliate in kind. How foolish we both were. How could we not have trusted in our love?* She remembered how despite themselves, eventually their love had won through, and how forgiveness had strengthened their resolve to nurture each other's needs, creating an even stronger love than they had had before.

She thought of how their love had grown over the years, as memories of the many adventures they had shared together with their little family spiralled through her mind. Sailing away from the country they had called home into the wide blue ocean, watching the familiar land disappear below the horizon. Seeing Glen strong and sturdy at the wheel, the concentration on his face as he glanced at the swinging compass, carefully plotting their course on the chart. The quiet and tranquil moments while bobbing about on the glassy water of a sea becalmed. The excitement of glimpsing the many sea creatures whose world they had entered, the beauty of a gliding shark, the unity of a school of tiny fish, the speed of a passing manta ray, and the stillness of a confused flying fish when it landed unintentionally on the deck. The comical look from the head of a tortoise, the smooth touch of a dolphin's skin and the depth of the gaze from the eye of a whale.

*

She felt again the strength of her man, young and vibrant, as he showed her how to trim the sails and steer the boat, holding a steady course. She recalled how he had sat little Joy on his lap and had shown her how to navigate with a sextant. She recalled how he had held his son's hand steady on the wheel as they sailed downwind through heavy seas, instilling his love of sailing forever in Scott's soul. She sighed as she remembered the stormy days and nights of raging seas and screaming winds, and how Glen's calm confidence had kept them going.

Scenes from a tropical paradise of coral atolls and windswept sandy beaches scrolled through her mind in picture postcard memories from their times on shore. Recalling their boat swinging at anchor in a protected harbour, she remembered how they had explored the many islands together; strolling hand in hand walking barefoot along the sand beneath the tall coconut palms; meeting and eating with the local people; watching their children play unabashed with the local children, their blond hair and fair skin causing much hilarity amongst their new friends.

She recalled the rare moments that they shared alone together, times when they first arrived at a new island and the people would come out to greet them, insisting on taking the children ashore in their canoes so they could rest and sleep before coming ashore later for a feast they had prepared for them. She chuckled to herself as she remembered how instead, they had made mad, passionate love before eventually rowing ashore and trying not to fall asleep during the feast!

*

"What are you thinking about?" Glen asked.

She shook herself back to the present and smiled. "You," she said, "I was thinking about you."

"Really?" he winked at her as he drove the car into their driveway and pulled to a stop. He reached over and took her hands in his. "You know I'll take care of you, no matter what," he said looking deep into her eyes. "We're in this together, for better for worse, remember?" He leaned forward and kissed her lightly on her forehead.

"Yes, I remember," she said, resting her head on his shoulder.

"OK then, let's eat," he said. "I'm hungry."

Ariena laughed and thought how much she loved this man she had come to know so well.

*

They didn't speak much during their meal, each lost in their own thoughts. As they finished eating, Ariena finally voiced her concern. "What if it's cancer?" she asked abruptly.

"What if it is?" Glen recounted.

"Well, what if they have to cut my breast off?" she said bluntly.

"Then I guess you'll be a little lopsided," he replied, smiling wanly at her.

"Seriously," she said, looking at him. "Will it make a difference?"

"Well, you'll probably walk around in circles for a while until you get used to it," he replied.

"You know what I mean," she said. "Will you still love me?"

Glen stood up and walked around the table, reaching his arms out to take her hands in his, and raising her to her feet, he pulled her to him. He wrapped his arms around her, holding her tightly. "Do you really need to ask me that?" he said as he released her enough to look into her eyes. "You know I'll always love you."

Tears welled in her eyes as she looked at his concerned face. "Yes, but, I mean, will you want to make love to me?" she asked.

"Hmm," he whispered into her hair. "I thought that might be what you were thinking," he said. He sat down and pulled her onto his lap. He took her face in his hands and gently turned it towards his, their eyes met and a tear escaped and rolled down her cheek. He scooped the tear and kissed the wetness on his finger, keeping his eyes locked in her gaze. "My darling, you know how much I love you and your beautiful body," he said smiling at her as she turned her head away and blinked back another tear. "There isn't any part of you I don't love from your fingertips to your toes and especially, I do love your breasts," he added mischievously. He took one hand from her cheek and with his thumb he tilted her chin towards him. His other hand wiped away a tear as his face became serious again. "If they cut your breast off, as you so delicately put it," he said, raising an eyebrow at her, "I will love you just the same," he said.

"Really?" she sniffed. "Do you really think so?"

He held her then and whispered in her ear, "I know so, my love, I know so."

She put her arms around him and buried herself in his embrace.

Wrapped in each other's arms, Ariena sobbed quietly as Glen stroked her hair. Eventually, as her sobs slowly abated, he whispered, "Feel better now?"

She nodded and sat upright, looking into his eyes she whispered, "I love you."

His face lit up with a loving smile and tapping her nose he said, "Now that's my girl." He winked at her and twirling her hair in his finger he said, "I was thinking, maybe I could kiss it better." The mischievous look had returned to his face.

\*

"Show me where this lump is and I'll take care of it," he said as he started to unbutton her blouse. As Ariena watched his fingers loosen the fabric of her shirt, she felt the undeniable tingle of arousal sweep through her. The shirt fell open and he gently pushed it off her shoulders and onto the floor. She hadn't worn a bra since burning it back in the sixties. Her breasts were round and full, hanging slightly on her chest, not pert and upright as they had been back then. Instead, they bore the swollen marks from years of breast feeding and tiny blue veins reached out towards the darkened colour around her nipples.

"It's here," she said, taking Glen's hand and placing it on her left breast. His fingers moved softly over her breast until he felt the hardness of the lump.

"There?" he said, pulling his fingers away as he touched it.

"I don't know," she answered. "I can't feel anything when you touch it."

"It doesn't hurt?" he asked.

"No," she replied, taking his hand again and placing it back on her breast.

"Well, in that case," he murmured, as he cupped her breast in his hand and kissed it softly.

"Hmmm, that makes it feel much better," she said, running her fingers through his hair as he bent over and kissed her breast again. Moving slightly, he brushed his lips over her nipple, running his tongue around it, the nipple rising to meet his lips as he kissed it again.

"I get the feeling it's still working too," he smiled as he took her face in his hands, slid his fingers through her hair, then pulled her towards him. He pressed his lips to hers, kissing her long and hard, his lips opening around hers, their saliva mixing as he slowly moved his tongue inside her mouth. She felt the thrill of his kiss race through her body, her heart throbbing in her chest, her breasts filled with a pleasurable ache as her nipples hardened, a piercing tingle shot from her breasts downward, bursting in an explosion of ecstasy and she felt the moistness between her legs. She gasped, closing her arms around his neck kissing the softness of his ear and whispered again, "I love you." Glen tightened his arms around her and carried her through the bedroom door, deftly kicking it shut behind them. He gently laid her on the bed, and looking into her eyes mouthed the words, "I love you too."

*

His hands slowly moved from her face across her shoulders and down her arms. He squeezed her hands and lifted her fingers to his lips, gently kissing her fingertips as he continued to look deep into her eyes. He placed her arms gently on the bed beside her body and slid his hands up to her breasts. Lowering his body over hers, he opened his mouth and sucked her nipples gently. Her body contorted under his as he ran his tongue around and over her nipples, licking the hardness of them. She moaned, arching her back to raise her breasts higher. He looked up and smiled at her, his whisper barely audible, "I love you."

His hands followed the contour of her body, down from her breasts and across her abdomen. He hooked his fingers in the top of her pants, slowly pulling them down. She pulled her feet up and lifted herself off the bed as he continued to remove her clothes, his eyes falling on her soft mound. He stooped and kissed her there briefly, with just enough pressure for her to feel his lips on her and for her body to respond with a tingling shudder. He let his own pants drop, kicking them onto hers. He took her feet in his hands and slowly lifted them to his mouth, kissing each toe lightly as she moaned with pleasure again. He lowered her feet and pulled his shirt over his head dropping it to the floor. Placing his hands back on her feet, he slowly moved them upwards and inwards, gently applying more pressure as he parted her legs enough for him to slide his naked body between them. She felt the warmth of his body envelope her as he lowered himself onto her, his hardness pressing into her abdomen as he brought his arms around her, lifting her slightly to kiss her forehead, her closed eyelids and the tip of her nose before lowering her again and placing his lips on hers. His tongue slipped easily into her mouth and she moved her lips with his, pushing her tongue into his mouth, tasting the sweetness of their kiss. He kissed her nose and eyes and neck. He gently nipped her earlobe, his teeth just touching enough to send another tingle of pleasure through her. He moved down her body, kissing the hot skin of her shoulders and chest, brushing his lips lightly over her erect nipples as he moved further down, kissing her abdomen and finally kissing the softness of her mound. She moaned with pleasure as his kisses sent another wave of tingling warmth through her.

\*

Raising himself to his knees, he traced his fingers over her mound, slowly moving inward to touch the wet softness within. He lowered his mouth onto her, kissing the soft folds of her skin, his tongue gently licking her hardness, his hot breath filling her with warmth. With a sudden rush of moisture, her body arched compulsively as she climaxed with shuddering pleasure. Her body shuddered again as he put his arms around her and pulled her to him. He wrapped his legs around hers and held her as deep sobs wracked her body. She buried her face into his neck and whispered between the sobs, "I love you, I love you," over and over again. He nuzzled her face with his and held her tightly, rocking her back and forth. As her sobbing slowed, he lowered her down onto the bed and pulled the sheets up over them. He kissed her wet cheeks and whispered softly, "Sleep now, my love."

\*

Ariena slept soundly for several hours before waking to find herself still wrapped in Glen's arms. She opened her eyes and looked towards him. In the darkness of the night, she could barely see the contours of his face. She moved closer and kissed his closed eyelids. He did not move. She kissed them again and he murmured, "Mmmm," as a smile flickered over his face. She gently kissed his smiling lips and his eyes fluttered open.

"You awake?" he said, kissing her lightly on the nose.

"Uh, huh," she said, raising herself above him.

"Come here," he said, reaching his arms out to her, pulling her down towards him. He tightened his arms around her and she felt his hardness against her.

"Hmmm," she whispered. "What about you?"

"Yep," he said, "I'm awake now." She smiled at him. Their lips moved together in a loving kiss. She felt the burning heat of him move deep inside her, filling her completely. She felt the pressure rising within her and the sudden mixture of heat and intense pleasure rush through her as her wetness flooded over him. He gasped as she felt him release into her, and parting from their kiss, he whispered, "I love you." She collapsed onto his warm body, nuzzling her face into his chest. He wrapped his arms around her and held her tightly. After a few minutes, he rolled her over onto her back. Looking into her eyes he said, "You'll be OK. Trust me. Whatever it is, there's nothing a little love wont take care of." He smiled mischievously again and added, "Imagine what a lot more love could do." He kissed her nose playfully and she laughed. They played lovingly, rolling back and forth, touching and kissing each other, until eventually sleep overtook them and they lay in each other's arms, content in the depth of their trust and love for each other.

# CHAPTER 3
## REALITY CHECK

The next morning, Ariena could not find the lump. She did the usual breast self-examination in the shower and found nothing. She specifically touched the area where she had found it the day before – not a trace of a lump. Her heart missed a beat, *Oh, thank God,* she thought, *it's gone.* She felt the welling in her chest and started to weep quietly. She stood longer in the shower, letting the soothing water wash away her tears and warm her body.

"Are you OK?" Glen asked when she entered the kitchen, humming a favourite tune as she sat down.

"Oh, yes, perfectly OK," she replied with a big smile. She looked at him and said triumphantly, "It's gone."

"What? Are you sure?"

"Yep, completely gone. Must have been just bruising after all," she stated. A worried look passed over Glen's face.

"Well, you *are* going to have it checked out though, right?"

"No need, there's nothing to check," she said, dismissing it while reaching for a piece of toast.

"It can't just disappear like that, can it?" he persisted.

"Maybe it was never there."

"I felt it too Ari, it was there. I don't know how it can disappear, but I think you should have it checked out just in case."

"Well, OK if it makes you happy," she said, leaning over and patting his hand.

"Good," he said, kissing her head, "I'd better get off to work."
She watched as he put on his jacket and reached for the door.

"Love you," he said, smiling and blowing her a kiss.

"Love you too," she replied, as the door closed behind him.
*What a guy*, she thought with a smile. She had no intention of
making an appointment to 'have it checked out just in case'.
"Probably wouldn't get an appointment today anyway. I'll leave
it a couple of days and think about it then," she said out loud to
herself, knowingly talking herself out of calling at all. She was
happy that the lump had gone and, although there was still a
tiny measure of doubt in her mind, she rejected it as being silly
and worrying unnecessarily. *If there really was a lump there*, she
thought, deliberately ignoring the fact that she had felt it herself,
*and if it is anything that needs checking out, then I'm sure I'll feel it
again. Meanwhile, no point in worrying over something that isn't
there*, she reasoned.

At that moment the phone rang, it was Joy calling to ask how
she was doing.

"Oh, great thanks sweetheart, how's the little one?" she asked,
hoping to steer the conversation away from discussing her.

"What's happening with you, Mum?" Joy asked, ignoring her
attempt at subterfuge.

"Oh that," she said, trying to sound casual. "Turned out to be
nothing after all, just bruising, nothing to worry about. Like I said
yesterday, your little man has quite the grip," she laughed. "What
are you up to today?" she asked, changing the subject.

"Well," Joy paused, "your *big* man has quite the grip on you too,"
she said. "Dad phoned to say he was concerned that you might
not make an appointment to have a checkup. He told me that you
couldn't find the lump this morning and that you didn't think it
necessary to have it checked out." She paused again before adding,
"So, I'm going with you to the appointment that I've made for you."

Ariena smiled in spite of herself. "OK," she sighed. "He knows me too well, but really, there is no lump there now," she added.

"The appointment is in an hour," Joy said. "Ill be there to pick you up in 30 minutes, be ready Mum."

"OK, OK," she said, "but I'm sure it will be a waste of time."

"Well, I hope so," Joy replied.

*

"From what you've told me," the doctor said, sitting down after having examined Ariena's breast, "and going by the fact that I cannot feel anything unusual in your breast tissue, I would say that you may have had what is commonly referred to as 'surfacing'."

"What does that mean?" Ariena asked.

"Well, it's a situation where there is a 'lump' present, but it is well below the surface tissue and would not normally be felt during self-examination, unless that is, it moves, or surfaces. Surfacing can occur for a number of reasons, but the most common is trauma to the tissue, such as what you described as occurring while holding your grandson."

"I wouldn't have called that trauma to the tissue," Ariena said. "I mean, it wasn't like a blow or anything like that," she reasoned, "and if this did occur, where's the lump now? Can it go back?" she asked.

"Trauma to the tissue is not necessarily traumatic at the time. It can occur over time as well, and yes, the lump can 'go back', as you put it," the doctor replied smiling at her.

"So, what do we do? Wait for it to surface again?" Ariena asked.

"No. Since there may be a lump present, it is best to try to identify what it is, sooner rather than later. Then if need be, we can do something about it."

"I hope you are not going to suggest I have a mammogram," Ariena said. "Now that would be trauma to the tissue, wouldn't it?" Doctor Dubois walked around the desk and pulled up a chair beside her. She took Ariena's hands in hers and looked at her steadily. "I know how you feel about mammograms," she said, "and as a woman, I'm inclined to agree with you, but as your doctor, I have to say that a mammogram may detect something that we can't manually. It can also identify the lump if it is detected." Ariena looked at her friend and sighed. "I know you have to recommend it Fran," she said, "but there must be other ways to detect a lump if it's there, that is not so traumatic? To the tissue I mean," she added. "I'm not concerned about the discomfort or pain of having a mammogram, it's just that it doesn't make sense to drastically traumatise the tissue to that extent," she reasoned. "What about an ultra sound? That is not so invasive. Would that detect the lump?"

"An ultra sound detects fibrous tissue," Fran replied, reverting to her professional manner. "So, if the lump is a cyst, it would show on the ultra sound."

"Right," said Ariena, "but what you are saying is that the ultra sound wont detect a non fibrous growth, like a tumour for instance?"

"Correct."

"Well, if I have an ultra sound at least we'd know if it was a cyst or not."

"Possibly. However, you do not have a history of cysts, nor do you have what is referred to as 'lumpy breasts'. Some women live with cysts and lumpy breasts and never have a problem."

"So, you're suggesting that in my case, the lump would more likely be a tumour."

"I'm suggesting that it would be a good idea to find out."

"Breast cancer," Ariena said bluntly. "It could be breast cancer."

*There, I've said it. The 'C' word.* She felt better getting it out in the open. *Lump and cyst, tumour and tissue just didn't have the same affect. Cancer, now there's a word with real affect. Especially if you put the word breast in front of it.*

"Ariena, we don't know that, that's why we need to do some tests. We need to know what we're dealing with." Her friend squeezed her hands and returned to the desk, resuming her professional status. "If you would rather have an ultra sound at this point, then let's at least do that. I also want you to have some blood tests done, I will make sure you can get in this afternoon," she said reaching for the phone.

*

Folding her arms across her breasts as if to protect them from what may ensue, Ariena sat listening to the phone conversation. She couldn't detect any concern in her friend's voice. *Must be hard to be two people at once,* she thought. *She's good though, at least I know I can trust her to tell me the truth.*

"That's good," her doctor said putting the phone down. "You can go there now and have the tests and ultra sound done immediately." She handed Ariena two slips of paper. "Hand those in when you get there and don't bother trying to read what I've written," she added with a smile. "I've got the doctor's handwriting down perfectly."

"Yes, I see that," Ariena agreed, looking at the professional scrawl on the paper. As she stood up she looked at her friend again and added, "Sorry to take so much of your time Doctor," she raised her eyebrow at the sign on the wall. "I've overextended my 10 minutes and definitely asked more than one question."

"That sign is not there for *my* patients," her friend said, giving her a quick hug. "I'll have my receptionist call you when I get the results of the tests so you can make an appointment and we'll discuss this further. Meanwhile, don't spend any time worrying about what might or might not be. Once we have the test results we'll be in a better position to know what we're dealing with. This may just be a reality check," she said with a smile.

"Yes, Doctor," Ariena returned her friend's hug. "Thanks for being you Francine."

# CHAPTER 4
## DIAGNOSIS

When the phone rang Ariena jumped. She'd been expecting it to ring, waiting more with trepidation than anticipation. She took a deep breath as she reached for the receiver. It was not her doctor's receptionist as she had expected, but the doctor herself.

"I have your test results and the ultra sound report," Dr Dubois said. "The results are not conclusive and I want you to have more done before you come in to discuss them."

"What is not conclusive, the blood tests or the ultra sound?" Ariena asked.

"Both. There is some indication from the blood tests that there may be a tumour present and the ultra sound does not show any abnormal fibrous tissue," the doctor replied. "To get a conclusive result we need to locate the tumour and identify its status."

"So, what further tests will do that?" Ariena asked, knowing what the answer would be.

"At this stage, I'm recommending that you have a mammogram to try to locate the tumour. If that is successful, we have more chance of identifying whether it is benign or malignant." Her friend's voice has taken on the serious tone of a professional doctor. She was no longer suggesting anything, she was recommending, which told Ariena that she was concerned. Before Ariena could say anything, Dr Dubois went on to explain further. "Once we have located the tumour, we can take a sample from it that is identified in the laboratory, the procedure is called a biopsy," she explained. "The pathologist's report will not only identify the nature of the tumour, but will also provide recommendations for further treatment if required. Without this information we have nothing to go on. The mammogram is the only technology we have that may be able to locate the tumour," she added. Ariena said nothing. The silence on the phone was deafening as the doctor waited for her reply.

"Ari?" her friend broke the silence. "Do you understand what I've said?"

"Yes, I heard you and I believe I understand what you are saying," she replied. "Do I have a choice?" she asked.

"You always have a choice, Ari," came the reply. "You can choose to do nothing at all and wait to see what transpires. However, without conclusive identification, you don't know whether time is of the essence here. In my professional opinion, that would not be a wise choice."

"OK," Ariena said with a sigh. "I know what the mammogram is, but tell me more about the biopsy. Does it require an anaesthetic?"

"No, the biopsy is like having a blood test, but with a needle that is a bit larger. It is inserted into the tumour to extract a sample of tissue. It can be a little uncomfortable and obviously there will be the pain of inserting the needle. However it doesn't take long, it's over in a few minutes."

"Seems to me extracting tissue would be a little more painful than extracting blood," Ariena commented. "Sounds like the definition of 'trauma to the tissue' to me," she added. The doctor said nothing. "It's not the pain that I'm concerned about," she continued. "I just don't like the idea of any procedures that will compromise the tissue further. It doesn't make sense to me." The doctor remained silent. "My instinct is telling me that there must be another way, but I don't know what it is," she went on. "I mean, if there is a problem and we were to identify the cause, then shouldn't we address that first?" she reasoned.

"If we haven't identified whether there is a problem, how can we identify the cause?"

"Well, we're assuming that there is a problem," Ariena stated. "What about diet? Is there something I should or shouldn't be eating that would make a difference?"

"There is no evidence that diet would have any affect on disease in the body," replied the doctor in a monotone. "There are no studies to indicate that diet has anything to do with health."

"That sounded like a standard answer Fran,' Ariena retorted.

"It was," her friend replied. "Ari, you can make changes to your diet if you want. I can only offer you advice and recommend what the medical profession has to offer in your circumstances. At this stage, to make any decisions as to a course of action if it is required, we need to determine what, if any, the problem is."

"I know, I'm sorry. I just think there must be a more natural approach to this, but I can't put my finger on it right now. It's like, I need more time to think. Do I need to make a decision right now on the mammogram and biopsy?"

"That would be preferable," Dr Dubois replied, sounding a little exasperated. "Once we have the results and pathologist report, you will know whether you need more time to think. There may not be anything to be concerned about." Ariena closed her eyes and took a deep breath. "OK," she said. "I'll do it. Let's get it over and done with." Fran's sigh was audible. "Good," she said, resuming her professional manner. "You have an appointment for the mammogram at 1 p.m. today and the biopsy is booked in for 3 p.m. tomorrow. I will receive the results of the mammogram in the morning and will phone you if there is any change to the biopsy appointment."

"You took the liberty of making the appointments without having my decision?" Ariena said.

"There are people lining up, Ariena. The waiting rooms are packed all the time," came the answer. "I don't want you to wait any longer than necessary," her friend explained. "If you don't hear from me in the morning, go to the biopsy appointment and my receptionist will let you know when to come in and discuss the results."

\*

*She was right,* Ariena thought. *There are people lining up. Something is very wrong with this picture.* She felt embarrassed that she was taken in immediately when she arrived. The mammogram went as predicted, a highly confronting experience. *Uncomfortable is not the word, feels more like I've been squeezed out of all proportion,* she thought. *Must have been invented by a man, bet they don't use it to identify testicular cancer,* she mused at the thought of how that would be achieved.

There was no phone call the next morning. By midday Ariena knew she would have to keep the biopsy appointment. She took a deep breath as she reached for the receiver. Her daughter answered her call. "I have to keep the biopsy appointment," Ariena said, swallowing a lump in her throat. "It means the mammogram located a tumour."

"Do you want me to come with you?"

"No, it's OK, thanks," she said. "You have the little one to take care of."

"You'll be fine, Mum," Joy said, trying to reassure her. "Call in on your way home for a cup of tea."

Ariena felt a wave of emotion sweep over her. "Thanks, sweetheart, I will," she said. Placing the phone down, she fought back the tears that were threatening to overtake her. *How blessed am I to have such a caring family,* she thought as she walked out the door.

*

*Francine was wrong,* Ariena thought. *That was nothing like having a blood test and the needle was not a bit larger, it was huge! A little uncomfortable? That's a joke. How many times did he insert the needle before he even started to extract the tissue? Five maybe, I lost count trying to stay calm.* She got into her car and looked at the clock. 'Doesn't take long,' Francine had said. 'Over in a few minutes,' she had said.

"I've been in there two hours!" Ariena said out loud. She reached up to adjust the rear view mirror, rubbing her arm unintentionally on her still tender breast. "Ow," she exclaimed. Looking at her reflection in the mirror she nodded. "I was right," she said, "I can still feel that tearing sensation. Wait till I see her!"

*

Her little grandson's face lit up with a big smile. "Nannie!" he cried with excitement, reaching his arms out for her to take him from her daughter. He gave her a big kiss and nuzzled into her chest. She winced as his little body pressed against her breast.

"Nannie got owie?" he asked, a little frown appearing on his forehead.

"Yes, darling. Nannie has got an owie," she said smiling at him.

"Kiss better?" Kenny buried his little face in her shirt and kissed her loudly. "Aw better," he declared and struggled to get down. Ariena lowered the boy to the floor, looking up at her daughter she smiled and said, "He's just like his Poppa! I wish it was that easy, little man," she patted him on the head as he rushed off to play with his toys.

"No fun, huh?" her daughter asked. "Sit down, I'll make some herbal tea, maybe chamomile to help calm you down?"

"Thanks, sweetheart. I should have had some beforehand! Not the funnest time I've ever had, that's for sure!" she commented wryly.

"So what now?"

"Have to wait for the results, could be a couple of weeks they said."

"…and meanwhile?"

"Meanwhile, I'm going to do some research," Ariena replied. "If it is cancer, then I want to know what the options are other than what I'm sure will be offered to me through the medical system," she added.

"Good idea," Joy agreed. "Better than sitting around worrying while you wait."

*

While Ariena sat in the waiting room she glanced around at the twenty or so people there. She thought about some of the research she had been doing. *If the ratio for breast cancer is 1 in 9, there are two people in this room that either have it, or are going to be diagnosed with it,* she thought. *It's like playing Russian roulette every time you sit amongst a group of people.*

Dr Dubois appeared in the doorway and waved her in. "How are you?" she asked, as Ariena entered the consulting room.

"I think you are about to tell me," Ariena said, raising her eyebrows at her friend.

"Yes, please sit down," she said, her professional manner immediately giving Ariena a hint of what was to come.

"It's bad news isn't it?" Ariena said, looking directly at her.

"It's not good news," Dr Dubois agreed. "The results of the biopsy show that the tumour is not benign," she said, looking down at the paper in front of her.

"Which means?"

"It's malignant."

"You mean, it's cancer."

"Yes, it's cancer." They sat silently looking at each other, Dr Dubois waiting for the gravity of the news to sink in. CANCER, cancer, cancer. The word seemed to reverberate around the room.

"It can't be," Ariena declared. "I'm healthy. I eat well and I'm physically fit. I'm not in pain," she added, "apart from having that biopsy you recommended," she said. "That was not amusing. Have you ever had a biopsy?" she asked. Not waiting for her friend to answer, she continued, "I felt sorry for the poor intern, he was so embarrassed. He must have tried five times with that needle before he found the tumour, and he was so apologetic each time. Seriously, he was talking to me as if I was already doomed, like he had read the pathologist's report already. Then it took forever to extract the tissue, and that was not uncomfortable," she exclaimed, glaring accusingly, "That was damn painful…"

"Ari, stop," Dr Dubois interrupted her outburst. "Calm down. I'm sorry about your experience with the biopsy," she said, "but it has given us conclusive results. Not the best, I grant you," she added, "but at least now we know what we're dealing with." She poured a glass of water for her friend and passed it to her. Ariena took the water. "Thanks," Ariena said, "you're right. I need to get my head around this, sorry," she muttered between sips.

"It's a perfectly natural reaction." Dr Dubois smiled at her. "Take time during the next few days to relax if you can. It's going to be a tough road ahead, you'll need to be in control of your senses and your emotions. As you said yourself, you are otherwise healthy and physically fit. You have a strong personality and a practical nature. If anyone can get through this, you can, but you will also need to take care of yourself," she said.

*

Ariena looked at her friend, the doctor she trusted to always tell her the truth. "How bad is it Fran?" she asked.

"The tumour is about the size of a golf ball, you need to have surgery to remove it. It may only require what is called a lumpectomy, removal of the lump or mass, the tumour. You have an appointment tomorrow with the surgeon, he will explain the procedure."

"How bad is it?" Ariena persisted.

"Ari," she said, reaching out her hand.

"Just tell me Francine, as a friend," Ariena said, "how bad is it?"

"It's bad," her friend said. "The cancer has been identified as being highly aggressive carcinoma, it is mutating rapidly and may have spread to the lymph nodes or further. They wont know for sure until during the surgery."

"Highly aggressive?" Ariena repeated the phrase. "Who makes these expressions up?" she asked no-one in particular. She looked at her friend's concerned face and saw the empathy in her eyes. "Sorry. You said it's spreading rapidly? How can that suddenly be the case?"

"It's not sudden Ari, this has been occurring for some time, possibly several years."

"Oh, great!" Ariena put her head in her hands and stared at the desk in front of her. The doctor waited in silence for the question she knew her friend would ask next. Ariena took a deep breath and looked up. "Am I going to die?" The question seemed to bounce around the room, trying to find an answer.

"We're all going to die eventually."

"Standard answer," Ariena retorted under her breath. "Let me rephrase that Doctor. How long have I got?" she said bluntly.

"I can't answer that question, Ari. I'm sorry. We wont know until after the surgery what the prognosis is," Dr Dubois replied, "and you will have to see the oncologist for that. An appointment at the Cancer Clinic will be made for a week after the surgery. Your test results, the pathologist's report and surgeon's report will be forwarded to the team of oncologists at the Cancer Clinic. They will discuss the diagnosis and will come to a collective decision as to their recommendations in your case. They will have appointed an oncologist to discuss that with you."

"Do you have any idea what their recommendations are likely to be?"

"No. As I said, that will depend on what they consider the prognosis to be."

"If they do recommend treatment, what do you think that would be?"

"Again, I can't answer that specifically. However, there are three types of treatment that are offered for breast cancer; surgery, chemotherapy and radiation. It will depend again on the prognosis whether chemotherapy and/or radiation are recommended after the surgery."

*

Ariena took another deep breath and let out an audible sigh. She stared at the blank wall, trying to take it all in. Her head was reeling, questions were spinning in and out of her mind. She didn't know which to ask first.

"Before you ask any more questions," her doctor said as if reading her mind, "allow me to make some suggestions. I understand that this is devastating news and it is hard to comprehend all the implications right now." She smiled at Ariena and continued. "Tomorrow the surgeon will discuss the surgery procedure with you so you will know what to expect there. Due to the nature of the cancer…"

"Highly aggressive," Ariena interrupted.

"Yes, highly aggressive, it is imperative that we move quickly. It is most likely that the surgery has already been booked at the hospital, probably by the end of this week, the surgeon will confirm this with you. I suggest you try to relax as much as possible during the next few days. I can recommend someone who can do reiki for you before, during and after the surgery, it will help tremendously with recovery," she added with a smile. "After the surgery, you will have a few days before your appointment with the oncologist. During that time you should write down all the questions that come to you. Write them in a book and take it with you to the appointment. There is transport available to you if you prefer not to drive there yourself. However I would suggest that you go with someone who will act as your advocate. Your husband, your daughter perhaps. It is best if someone goes with you as it will be difficult to comprehend and remember everything that is discussed. Your advocate can take notes during your discussion with the oncologist so you can refer to them afterwards, which will help with your making decisions at that stage."

"Good advice, thanks," said Ariena. "However, I do have one question for now. Is it absolutely necessary to have the surgery?"

"We have established that time is of the essence, Ari. The cancer is rapidly multiplying. Removing the tumour will at least slow the process down."

"I understand that, and the theory behind eliminating the cause," Ariena replied, "but the tumour is not the cause, is it? It's the result. My body has been compromised in some way that has caused the cancer to develop. Surely if we identify the cause and eliminate that, the cancer will stop multiplying. Surely then the tumour will shrink and die, so to speak?" The doctor said nothing. "Isn't there some other less invasive way than surgery to remove the tumour?"

"Not that we can recommend," her doctor answered. "Nothing that is proven scientifically." Ariena ignored the doctor's flat statement.

"The body must be able to reverse the situation, given the means," Ariena expressed her thoughts out loud. "I need to identify the cause." She looked at her doctor and saw sympathy in her friend's eyes. "I need more time to think about this," she said to her.

"You must discuss that with the surgeon tomorrow."

"Yes, I will," Ariena replied with a wan smile.

\*

"I'm sorry for my outburst earlier," Ariena said apologetically. "I realise you are in a difficult position, being that you're my doctor and we're also friends. Thanks for putting up with me, I'm sure other patients are not so highly aggressive," she said in an attempt at ironic humour.

"Like I said, as a doctor I consider it a perfectly natural reaction," her doctor replied. "As a friend though, I'm not so sure I will tolerate it." Her rejoinder at humour made them both laugh. "Remember," she added, "I am your friend first, your doctor second. I'm here for you as both." She stood and handed Ariena a slip of paper. "This is your surgeon's appointment time and the Cancer Clinic details. Also the contact for the reiki practitioner. You can of course, phone me at home anytime." Ariena took the paper and put it in her pocket. "Thank you," she said. The two friends smiled at each other. There was nothing more they could say.

# CHAPTER 5
## FEAR

Ariena walked past the people sitting in the waiting room wondering which one of them was the other statistic. She had played the game of Russian Roulette and had lost. The bullet was firmly lodged in her brain, manifesting as the word that had just changed her life forever. She tried to clear her thoughts, but the voice in her mind kept saying that word cancer, cancer, CANCER. She pushed the heavy glass door open and stepped outside in a daze. The door slowly closed behind her and in the last second slammed shut. That was exactly how she was thinking about her life: fifty years slowly closing behind her and the last few seconds slamming shut.

*

Her head was spinning and she faltered in her step. Reaching out, she steadied herself against a tree. The rough bark on the tree trunk felt reassuringly alive. She wanted to put her arms around the tree and hold on for dear life. Tears welled up and she blinked them away. She let go of the tree, wiped her eyes and walked slowly towards her car. Fumbling through her bag, she pulled out several items before finally recognising the clink of the keys. She opened the door, threw her bag onto the passenger seat, climbed in and sat staring straight ahead through the windscreen. Her eyes saw nothing, her mind reeled in a swirling haze of fog. Through the fog, the words kept coming at her. Faster, louder:

cancer, cancer, CANCER, they burst into her consciousness, penetrating her mind, her body and her very soul.

\*

Ariena suddenly felt the overwhelming need to get away, far away from this place where the words were coming from. She turned the key in the ignition and the car's engine started humming. Like an automated robot, she shifted the gear lever into reverse and without looking in the rear vision mirror backed the car out of the parking space. She shifted into forward gear and drove out onto the road, looking neither left nor right, she gave way to no-one. A surprised driver in an oncoming car, braked to avoid hitting her, then leaned on his horn. She didn't see or hear him.

Somehow she managed to drive through the town and out into the countryside without causing an accident. Once on the open road, her mind cleared and reality slowly started to kick in. *Oh my God, what am I going to do?* The car hurtled on down the road, picking up speed as her foot pressed hard against the accelerator, her eyes staring at the long straight road ahead, the knuckles on her hands turning white as they gripped the steering wheel. Fleeting images of the scenery flashed past as she blithely pressed on. A slight curve in the road ahead brought her suddenly back to the present, she glanced at the speedometer, the needle wavering at 120 kilometres per hour. Taking her foot off the accelerator, slowing the car slightly before reaching the curve, then accelerating again as she drove around the corner, she took control of the car and herself.

Once through the corner, Ariena looked for a place to pull over. Not far ahead there was a small rest area off to the side of the road. She drove in, parked and turned off the ignition. *Whoa! Close encounter of another kind! Good thing there was no other traffic on the road, she thought, especially no traffic cop! I'm sure I was just a tad over the speed limit.* Then another thought occurred to her: *Still, what could they do to me now? Fine me? Take my car away? Can't take my life away, that's been done!* The thought shocked her. It brought her back to the harsh reality of her situation. One that had not existed until a few hours ago. The doctor's words no longer pounded in her brain, the sudden realisation of how fragile life is, hit her with an even greater force.

*

Her body shook with an involuntary shudder. The thought of 'someone walking over her grave' was too close to bear. She felt the unmistakable welling in her gut as her stomach turned over. Quickly, she opened the car door and leaned out as her body convulsed into uncontrollable retching. Vomit hit the road and splashed back onto the car door, the acrid smell and taste of bile making her retch again. Tears squeezed out of her tightly closed eyes and ran down her cheeks. She moved to wipe them and felt the welling sensation overtake her again as she gagged and dry retched, three times in rapid succession. Her stomach fluttered once, then the feeling subsided. She sat back in the seat, panting from the sudden exertion. She reached over and pulled a tissue from inside her bag, wiped her mouth and made a disinterested attempt at wiping the door before shutting out the sight and smell of vomit. Her throat felt like she had swallowed a ton of razor blades. She reached for her water bottle and took a gulp of water, swished it around in her mouth, opened the door and spat it out. Another rinse made her throat feel a little better, she closed the door and sat back with an exhausted sigh.

*

Then her mind went blank. Shivers ran up and down her spine and she felt cold, even though it was a warm day. Her body started shaking. Wrapping her arms around herself, she bent over and tucked her chin in, lowering her head to her chest. Gulping sobs wracked her body as she opened her mouth and let out a long wail of anguish. Tears flowed into her mouth, the acridity of lingering vomit mingling with the salty taste. Her shoulders shook with the intensity of her crying. She couldn't stop and abandoning herself to the sheer force of it, she kept crying, momentarily shocking herself at the loudness of the wailing coming from her. She knew the sound was coming from deep within her soul. Deep sobs continued to wrack her body, leaving a dull ache in her chest. Finally she let out a scream of "No-o-o-o-o-o-oh!" followed by several low sobs that dissipated into a sound like that of a mother keening over the devastating loss of a child.

Eventually she sat up, wiped her eyes and her chin with the back of her hand and looked in the mirror. Her swollen eyes were red and puffy, her face blotched and crusty where the tears had dried. A few specks of vomit still clung to her bottom lip. She licked at it with her tongue and immediately wished she hadn't. "What a mess," she muttered. "Why me?" she asked her reflection. She stared blankly at herself, transfixed by her image in the mirror. How could she not have an answer to her own question? What was holding her back? As she stared into the mirror, she suddenly saw the answer reflected in her eyes. Fear! It was raw unadulterated fear. The realisation hit her with a palpable force. She covered her eyes with her hands, not wanting to see her image wracked with fear. She cowered into the seat, her body shrinking into the fetal position…

\*

Suddenly her body convulsed. Her eyes snapped open and she grasped for the door, as bile coursed up her throat, forcing her to retch yet again. *So that's what fear tastes like,* Ariena thought wryly as she wiped her mouth. Turning back to the mirror, she shook her head. "Anything that tastes that bad can't be good for you," she said purposefully, "so let's just eliminate it entirely, there's no room for fear in your life." She nodded in agreement with herself and slowly smiled at her image. A wave of relief washed over her, lifting her spirits and her resolve. "I can do this, I can eliminate fear completely from my life." She looked into her eyes and watched as a look of determination replaced the fear. "This is it," she told herself, "this is the biggest challenge you've ever faced and you've got to meet it head on, take control of your own life and give it all you've got." She banged the steering wheel with her fist, confirming her resolve. "Yes, I can do it, I can beat this thing." She looked back in the mirror and winked at herself. "Cancer?" she said, "No fear!"

*

Ariena turned the car radio on and a song blared out, "...*you are the best thing in my life*..." She nodded to herself. "Well, now that's over with, lets go deal with the rest. No more fear, we're leaving that behind." Ariena drove out onto the road, carefully checking her rear vision mirrors this time. Each time she caught a glimpse of herself in the mirror, she raised her eyebrows and smiled. She joined in the tunes on the radio singing aloud.

# CHAPTER 6
## SUPPORT

When Ariena arrived home, she found her mother busy in the kitchen and her father merrily shuffling plates around the table.

"Hello, what's going on here?" she said as she walked into the room. Her mother wiped her wet hands on her apron and held them out to hug her daughter. "You've been so busy with seeing doctors and all, we thought we'd come over and get dinner," she said. "How are you dear?" she asked, patting Ariena's cheek, searching her face for clues.

"I'm OK, Mum," Ariena lied. "What's for dinner?" she asked, changing the subject. Her mother took the hint and kissing her daughter lightly on the cheek, she stepped back to the sink. "I'm just finishing the salad and I've made your favourite, veggie lasagne. It's still in the oven, another 20 minutes and it will be ready," she announced looking through the oven door.

"What have you been up to today?" her father asked, as he selected a handful of cutlery from the drawer. Her mother patted his arm and said, "Not now, dear," shaking her head. He looked at the cutlery in his hand and then at his wife with a confused expression.

"Go ahead, finish setting the table, Ari will tell us about her day when she's ready," she said.

"Oh, right." He winked at his daughter.

Ariena laughed. "You're both so sweet," she said, "thank you for being here today, and making dinner," she added. She knew they were worried, but she wasn't ready to break the news just yet.

*

The door opened and a huge bunch of flowers appeared.

"TA, dah," Glen shouted as he came through the door, holding the flowers up high.

"Oh, young man, you shouldn't have," Ariena's mother said jokingly. "How lovely!" Glen bent over and kissed Ariena on the head. "They're for you, darling," he whispered, placing the flowers on her lap.

"What's going on?" Ariena's father asked, looking confused again.

Ariena laughed. "Thank you," she whispered to Glen, smelling the perfume of the flowers. She stood up and reached for a vase to put them in. "Mum's made dinner, it's almost ready," she said raising her eyebrows at him.

"OK, great!" he replied, "I'll be right with you." Ariena arranged the flowers in the vase and placed them on the table.

"Ah, that's what it needed'" her father said, "how'd he know?" Smiling, she kissed her father's cheek and said, "There, your job's done, Dad. Have a seat while I help Mum with the food."

*

"Great dinner, dear," Ariena's father said appreciatively, helping himself to another serving.

"Yes, this is delicious, Mum. I think it might be the best lasagne you've made. Salad is good too," Glen agreed, complimenting his mother-in-law.

"Well, I'm glad you boys are enjoying it," she said. "What about you dear," she turned to Ariena, "you're not eating much, not very hungry?"

"It is delicious, Mum," Ariena smiled at her mother. "It's just that I'm thinking I'm going to miss your cooking. You see, I may not be eating this kind of food in the future. So, I'm taking it slowly and enjoying every mouthful." Her mother looked at her questioningly but said nothing more as they continued their meal.

*

"Well, I guess I have something to tell you all," Ariena said once everyone had finished eating. "I didn't want to say anything before dinner and ruin the meal. It was lovely, Mum. Thank you both for being so thoughtful," she added, patting her parents' hands.

"Good food is meant to be enjoyed together with your family," her father said, nodding with a smile. He reached for the empty plates and started stacking them.

"Leave them, dear," her mother said to him, putting her hand on his and leaving it there.

"I love you all so much," Ariena blurted out, tears welling up in her eyes.

"Oh, shit!" Glen exclaimed, getting up to put his arms around her. "Sorry, Mum," he said, apologising to his mother-in-law for his language.

"I'm sorry," Ariena said, "I thought I had it under control. I thought I could tell you without blubbering again. I thought I'd already cried it all out," she said through her sobs.

"What's wrong, sweetheart?" her father took her hand in his and patted it. "Tell your old dad all about it. Nothing's too bad we can't fix it." Her mother squeezed his arm, smiling at him as tears rolled down her own cheeks.

"I've got cancer," Ariena said with finality. "I'm sorry, I don't know how else to say it." She gulped back a sob. "They've booked me in for surgery in two days."

"Shit," Glen said again without apology. "Oh, baby, no." He buried his face in her hair, kissing her repeatedly. Her mother put her hand on his shoulder. "Sit down, son," she said gently, "let her breathe." She stood up and reached for the kettle. "I'll make us all a nice cup of tea," she announced, making a brave attempt to stay calm herself as she wiped away her own tears with the back of her hand.

"That's a good idea, a nice cup of tea always helps when you're feeling down," her father said as he stood up to get the teacups.

*

"What did the doctor say, dear?" her mother asked as she poured the tea. Ariena sniffed and cleared her throat. "Well," she hesitated, still unsure how to say it. "There's a lump, a tumour that needs to be removed. That's what the surgery is for," she said.

"That's what little Kenny found?" her father asked.

"Yes, and a good thing he did too," Ariena replied. "Otherwise we might not have known it was there. Apparently it's been growing for a while, but they say it's still growing and might be spreading, so that's why they want to do the surgery."

"So, it's like exploratory as well as removing the tumour?" her mother suggested.

"Yes, they'll be looking to see if the cancer has spread anywhere else," Ariena replied. "I have an appointment with the surgeon tomorrow, I guess he'll explain it further then."

"Did the doctor say how, um, bad it is?"

"She said it is bad," Ariena replied flatly. "It's called highly aggressive, medical jargon for growing rapidly. That's why they want to do the surgery immediately, to slow it down."

"While they figure out what to do next?"

"I guess so." They all took a sip of their tea and said nothing.

*

Suddenly the phone rang, breaking the silence and making them all jump.

"I'll get it," her mother said, hopping up and leaving the room. Ariena took a deep breath and sighed. Her body shuddered involuntarily. She put both hands around the teacup as if to warm herself, but she wasn't cold. Just shattered. The two men looked over their teacups at her, not knowing what to do or say. Her father looked relieved as her mother returned. "Who was that dear?" he asked.

"Your granddaughter," she replied with a smile.

"How is she?"

"She's fine. She said to say hello and that she'll be around tomorrow when Kenny wakes up." She turned to Ariena and said, "She is going to put a call in to tell Scott your news. It's late there, so she'll leave a message for him to phone you tomorrow."

"Thanks, Mum," Ariena said, dreading the thought of having to tell her children herself.

*

Ariena's mother looked at her son-in-law and saw that he was staring blankly into space. She put her hand on his shoulder saying, "You two go and sit down in the living room while Dad and I do the washing up." She raised her eyebrows at her husband, who immediately jumped up and started clearing the table. "Yep, off you go," he said. "We can take care of these."

45

"Thanks, Mum," Ariena said again, getting up and kissing her mother. "You too, Dad," she smiled kissing him as well.

"Don't you worry about a thing," her father told her. "Nothing's so bad it can't be fixed," he repeated, "and don't bother coming out to see us off, we know the way out." He winked at her and patted his son-on-law on his back, giving him a gentle push. "Off you go, then."

*

Ariena and Glen sat on the couch holding hands and saying nothing. They could hear the dishes being washed up and put away. Eventually, they heard the back door open and close, and the car pull out of the driveway.

Ariena broke the silence with another deep sigh and leaned her head against Glen's chest. He wrapped his arms around her and whispered, "Oh my darling, darling girl." Tightly, he held her, resting his face on the top of her head. "We'll get through this, baby," he said, "and we'll come out the other side OK, you'll see. We always have and we always will." She nodded, but didn't say anything. She didn't want to speak anymore, she just wanted to stay in his arms like that forever. He put his hand under her chin and tilted her face towards him. He kissed her tear stained cheeks and looked at her sad face. "Oh, darling, you're exhausted," he said. "How about a nice hot bath," he suggested. "You lie down here and relax while I run the water for you." He gently lowered her head onto a cushion, and lifted her legs onto the couch. "Don't move, I'll be back for you when it's ready," he said leaving the room.

*

Ariena closed her eyes and tried to relax. She really did feel completely exhausted. *All that crying sure takes it out of you,* she thought. She could hear the water running into the bath. It was a comforting sound. She could hear her husband walking back and forth from the bathroom to the kitchen and into the bedroom. She wondered absently what he was up to. Then the scent of lavender wafted into her nose and she smiled. *Wonderful, he's found the lavender oil,* she thought as she dozed off.

The tap squeaked as the water was turned off, waking Ariena from her sleep. Glen walked into the room, dressed in his bathrobe and holding hers. "I almost dropped off to sleep," she said smiling at him as he kneeled down beside her.

"Yes, you're tired, and no wonder," he said. "That's why I'm going to give you a relaxing bath and get you to bed, it's been a long day." He kissed her on the nose and said, "Don't move, I'll get you undressed and into that bath, relax and leave it all to me." He kissed her lightly on the lips. "Gorgeous girl," he murmured, undoing her shirt and slipping it off her shoulders. He put his hands gently under her bare breasts and kissed each one. "Don't you worry," he said looking at them, "I'm going to take care of you too." Wrapping the bathrobe around her shoulders he pulled Ariena to her feet. "Come on," he said, lifting her over his shoulder, "let's get you in that bath." As he lowered her down to the floor beside the bath, he gently slid her pants down to her feet. Turning her around and slipping the bathrobe off her shoulders he said, "In you get."

Ariena gasped with surprise as she looked into the bath. The steam rose up from the water bringing with it the relaxing smell of lavender. Oil droplets floated on the water amidst a layer of rose petals. Two candles dimly lit the room, the flame light dancing on the walls and ceiling.

"Oh, it's beautiful," she exclaimed, turning to thank him.

"In you get," he repeated with a smile. "You lie down in there and relax for a while, then I'll join you and we'll wash away all those tears." Glen kissed her lightly on the lips again and held her hand while she stepped into the water. Sliding down amongst the rose petals she sighed, "It's delicious," she said, closing her eyes and soaking in the relaxing heat and aroma.

"Keep your head above water," he said jokingly, "I'll be back in a little bit."

She opened her eyes as he left the room, watching the rose petals floating over her body. *He's such a darling*, she thought. *Fancy him thinking of this, it's so lovely.* She chuckled as she noticed her nipples poking up above the water, the rose petals gently touching as they floated by. "Like as if you're not getting all the attention right now," she said.

"Who are you talking to?" Glen asked, returning to the room.

"My breasts," she said, laughing.

"Ah, yes," he laughed with her. "May I join you and your breasts?" he asked as he took his bathrobe off.

"That would be lovely," she answered, sitting up and making room for him. He stepped in and slid down behind her, wrapping his legs on either side of hers. Putting his hands on her breasts, he slowly lowered them both down into the water.

They lay there for a while, soaking in the warmth and ambiance. Eventually he whispered in her ear, "Let's get you washed before the water gets too cold." They sat up, and lathering the soap in his hands, he gently rubbed her body, covering her with tiny suds. Cupping his hands in the water, he poured handfuls of rose petals all over her, washing off the soap and leaving her adorned with the flowers. "Gorgeous girl," he said again, as he stepped out of the bath, lifting her to her feet. He wrapped the bathrobe around her and held her hand as she stepped out of the bath and into his arms. He pulled her to him, wrapping the bathrobe around them both as his arms encircled them. Their lips met, a long, slow enchanting kiss held them together, rose petals soft on their wet, oil enriched skin. They both sighed as the kiss ended.

"Come," he said, taking her by the hand and leading her to the bedroom. "It's time for your massage." She raised her eyebrows at him. "Really?" she said as she followed him. A faint smell of burning incense reached her as she entered the candle lit room. Glen stepped aside so Ariena could see the bed, covers pulled back and rose petals covering the sheet and pillow.

"Oh, my goodness," she exclaimed, and threw herself into his arms. "I love you!" He kissed her again as he gently picked her up and laid her on the bed. She returned his kiss, murmuring softly, "Mmm, so romantic!"

He took her face in his hands and whispered, "I love you too, so much, and tonight my love, you get to relax completely." He reached for the bottle of lavender oil beside the bed. "What you need is a deep, relaxed sleep," he said smiling at her. "So, I'm going to give you a deep, relaxing massage until you fall asleep. All you have to do is lie still and close your eyes." He leaned forward and gently closed her eyes with his fingers, lightly kissing both eyelids.

"Mmm," she sighed, keeping her eyes closed.

"Shhh," he whispered. She felt him move slightly and heard the sound of music softly fill the air. She smelt the swirling scent of lavender and felt the soothing touch of his hands massaging the oil deep into her skin, completely relaxing her mind, body and soul. As sleep enveloped her, Glen lay down beside her, and pulling the covers over them, he wrapped his arms around her, holding her safe in the warmth of his love.

\*

Deep in the recesses of her mind, Ariena heard a faint ringing sound. As the sleep drifted from her, she opened her eyes and recognised the sound. Carefully she extracted herself from the loving arms around her and slipped from the bed, grabbing her bathrobe as she went through the door. She picked up the telephone receiver and slurred a sleepy, "Hello?"

Her son's voice crackled through the line, "Mum? Is that you?"

"Yes," she answered, "hold on a moment, love." She quickly stepped back and closed the bedroom door. "Sorry, just closed the door, your Dad's asleep."

"Oh-oh, I forgot about the time difference," her son said. "Is it really late there?"

"No, it's really early," she said with a chuckle. "How are you Scott?"

"I'm fine. The question is, how are you Mum?"

"I'm fine too," she said, "for now. I guess you got the news?"

"Yes, we got the message a couple of hours ago. Mia and I have been arranging leave from work and getting flights," he said. "We can't come together, but I'll be there next week. Mia's flight is not for a couple of weeks after mine, but we can both stay till after Christmas," he said.

"Oh, darling, you don't have to come out," Ariena said. "We don't even know the full details, I haven't seen the surgeon yet."

"All the more reason for me to come out," her son replied. "The more support you have with you through this the better."

"That's very sweet of you dear, but…"

"No buts, Mum," he interrupted. "Our flights are booked and we're coming. I arrive on Wednesday, can't remember the exact time or flight number, I'll phone again tomorrow to give you the details so someone can pick me up."

"OK, it will be lovely to have you here," she said. "Do you mean you'll phone tomorrow or today? I think it's already morning, I can't quite see the clock from here."

"Don't worry, I'll phone Joy, she'll let you know. Now I better let you get back to bed before Dad finds you gone. Sneak back and have a sleep-in," he said with a laugh.

"Thanks, darling," she said, "I'm looking forward to seeing you."

"Me too, Mum. Now you take care and say hi to Dad for me when he wakes up. I'll see you soon, OK?"

"Yes, love, see you soon." Ariena put the phone down and pulled the robe around her. She felt cold as she walked back to the bedroom and slipped under the covers, snuggling up close to the warm body sound asleep in the bed. Glen's arm wrapped itself around her and he whispered, "How's Scott?"

"I thought you were asleep," she said, snuggling closer. "He's coming out next week and Mia's coming a couple of weeks later."

"Good lad," he said, tightening his arm around her. "The more support you have the better."

"That's what he said," she murmured, closing her eyes. "Hold me, I'm cold." Glen felt her body relax as sleep overtook her. He wanted to wipe the tears from his eyes as they trickled down his cheeks, but he couldn't let go of her. Holding her close in his arms, he whispered into her hair, "I wont let you go," and silently he wept.

# CHAPTER 7
## DENIAL

Ariena sat in the surgeon's waiting room looking at the rows of patient files on the shelves behind the receptionist's desk. She started counting them in blocks of ten to take her mind off why she was there. The receptionist took a file from the shelf and walked into an adjoining room, leaving the door ajar. *Oh my God,* Ariena almost voiced her thought aloud, as she saw the room was lined with shelves, all stocked full with more files. *There must be thousands,* she thought to herself. The receptionist walked out, closing the door on the thousands of stories. *I wonder if the files in that room are closed, like a morgue of faceless people?* The thought made Ariena shudder.

Reaching up and pulling another file from the shelf behind her, the receptionist called out the name written on the front. A woman in the waiting room stood and followed the receptionist into a smaller waiting room. Her file was placed in a pocket on the outside of the door.

"The doctor will see you shortly," the receptionist said as she closed the door. She went back to her desk and pulled another file. She repeated the process, this time a much younger woman, trailing two little children, was closed inside a small room, her file left upright in the pocket on the door. The receptionist pulled another file. Ariena looked around the waiting room at the people still sitting there. They all looked up expectantly. The next woman who was called had an anxious look on her face as the door closed on her. The receptionist sat down and busied herself at her desk, straightening a stack of papers, pushing a pot of pens to one corner, moving the phone to the other corner. Appearing satisfied, she sat back in her chair and reached for the cup of coffee sitting next to the computer. She took a sip, replaced the cup on the desk and stared at the computer screen.

*Feels like I'm watching a bad horror movie,* Ariena thought, *except this is for real! This is not normal. How come no-one else has noticed how bizarre this is?* she wondered. *Perhaps they've all been in this scene before.*

\*

Her thoughts were interrupted as the doctor's consulting room door opened and a teary-eyed woman walked out. Ariena caught a glimpse of the doctor sitting behind his desk as the door closed. The woman sniffed loudly as she walked through the waiting room, oblivious to everyone there. She handed her file to the receptionist and said nothing as she went out onto the street. Ariena watched her through the window. The woman appeared confused, not sure of where she was going. Ariena looked at the receptionist who remained at her desk, appearing unconcerned as she took another sip of her coffee. The woman was still standing on the pavement outside, alone in her despair. Ariena swallowed the lump in her throat. *I know exactly how she feels,* she thought. She looked at the woman again and wanted to go outside to give her a hug, but she also knew that comfort was not what this woman needed the most. *She needs to rid herself of the fear that has a hold on her,* Ariena thought. *I hope she can throw it up on her way home,* she thought wryly.

\*

The receptionist put down her coffee cup and walked to the first room, taking the file from the door as she opened it. "The doctor will see you now." Ariena watched as one followed the other towards the doctor's consulting room. The receptionist walked in and handed the file to the doctor, who remained seated. The woman who had followed sat down nervously in the chair facing the doctor. The receptionist closed the door and returned to her desk. Picking up a file she resumed the previous scene. Without so much as a glance toward the people in the waiting room, she called Ariena's name and started walking towards the now empty smaller waiting room door.

*She's like a robot*, Ariena thought to herself as she stood up to follow. *I wonder what would happen if I changed the script mid-scene?* "Can you show me the bathroom please?" she asked. The receptionist stopped walking and stood quite still for a second before turning to look at her. She had a look of sheer disbelief and shock.

*Ha, got you*, Ariena thought to herself while smiling sweetly.

"Ah, yes, of course," the receptionist answered. She pointed in the opposite direction. "It's down the hallway, first on the right. Please return to reception when you're done," she added.

"Thank you," Ariena said, still smiling as she walked past her. *Wonder what she's going to do with my file now*, she mused. Once in the bathroom she looked in the mirror and chuckled. "That threw her off, didn't it," she said to her reflection. "Well, at least I turned the horror movie into a comedy for a moment, wonder if the others even noticed." She chuckled again. *Wonder where else I could go other than reception after I'm done?* "Better get it over and done with," Ariena whispered to her reflection as she left the bathroom.

The receptionist had not moved and was still holding Ariena's file.

*Pick up where we left off, shall we?* Ariena thought still smiling sweetly as she approached. The receptionist turned and resumed the previous scene, placing her file in the door and delivering the one-liner: "The doctor will see you shortly."

"Incredible," Ariena said aloud as the door closed on her.

*

She looked around the small room, taking in the posters covering the walls. Posters of various views and angles of a woman's breast, depicted with and without skin and tissue. Cross section drawings showing the intricate weave of veins and milk ducts. A coloured picture of a nipple and areola, labeled in red. *So this is the part where you get familiar with the clinical breast,* Ariena thought. *Nothing beautiful or sensual here, just another body part. A piece of flesh, nothing more.* She looked around the rest of the room, half expecting to see a plastic model of a breast that came apart so you could see inside, but the room was relatively bare: one chair beside a shelving unit with a few technical books and a round glass paper weight. For a moment she thought it was in the shape of a breast, but it was not. *That would really be creepy, perfect for the horror movie though,* she mused. She sat down and stared at the empty top shelf. She tried to relax, but in her mind's eye she saw row upon row of glass jars with breasts inside, each labeled with a name. She shook her head and looked at the door, there was no window to look out and distract herself. The wood grain of the door swirled around tiny dots and dark knots, *veins, milk ducts, nipples.* She looked back at the empty shelf. Her imaginary glass jars became larger, the breasts inside floating, fleshy in a pale blue liquid. Some of the breasts were cut open, their eery insides visible. As she sat transfixed by the imagery, labels appeared on the jars: 'aggressive,' 'inverted,' 'unremarkable,' then below the labels on every jar, another label appeared, 'deceased.' "Oh, my God," she said aloud, standing up and taking a step towards the door. "I have to get out of here." The door swung open.

"The doctor will see you now." The receptionist marched towards the consulting room, holding her file. *No wonder those poor women looked so drained,* Ariena thought to herself, thankful to be leaving the room and following the receptionist just like the others had.

*

The doctor took the file from the receptionist and waved Ariena towards the chair without looking at her. She waited until the receptionist had left and shut the door before saying, "I'd rather stand for the moment if you don't mind Doctor Schwartz," she said, waiting for him to acknowledge her presence.

"Suit yourself," he replied, closing her file and looking at her. "You have been diagnosed with highly aggressive carcinoma, evident in the left breast," he announced. "This requires immediate surgery to remove the offending tumour. This procedure is expected to slow down or possibly arrest the cancer growth." Without waiting for a response from Ariena, he continued, "I will determine during the surgery whether the cancer has spread to the lymph nodes, in which case I will remove all the lymph nodes affected. This usually requires a second incision closer to the armpit, but with the location of the identified tumour it may be possible to perform both procedures through the one incision. However, depending on the amount of growth, it may also be necessary to remove the entire breast," he added.

Opening her file he announced, "Your surgery has been booked for this Wednesday at 8 a.m. You need to be at the hospital by 6.30 a.m. to complete the paperwork and be prepared for the surgery.

You can sign the consent form here," he said, pushing a paper form across the desk towards her.

Ariena reached for the back of the chair to steady herself. She felt her knees caving in, threatening to give way. She slowly lowered herself into the chair, attempting to appear unshaken. She collected herself and looked directly at the doctor. "Did you say that you may also remove the entire breast?" she asked.

"That is correct,'" he answered. "If it is evident during this surgery that removal is required, then it will be done immediately." Ariena looked at the doctor incredulously. "So, what you are saying is that *you* will decide whether to remove my breast during surgery," she stated.

"Yes," he replied without further explanation. Ariena let the full affect of what he had said register in her brain. "I don't think so," she said slowly, continuing to look directly at him. He looked up and held her gaze. "You're in denial," he declared. Waving his hand, he added, "Perfectly normal. It's hard for you to believe that you have cancer. I see from your doctor's notes that you are physically active and lead a healthy lifestyle. However, the fact remains that you do have cancer in a state of rapid growth, and we need to do what we can immediately to stop that growth. It's perfectly normal," he repeated, "for you to feel that your body has betrayed you, and considering your current state of health, it's normal for you to be in denial about having cancer."

"Denial, betrayal?" Ariena raised her voice slightly as she repeated his words.

"Yes, you're in denial, but that's all right," the doctor said, attempting to calm her. "You don't need to worry about anything, I'll decide during the surgery what needs to be done for the best." Glancing briefly at his watch, he picked up a pen and placed it on the form in front of her. "All you have to do is sign here," he said tapping the X marked on the form. Ariena sat forward in her chair, reached for the pen and twirled it around in her fingers.

*

"Just a minute," she said. "I need to get this straight. By signing this form I give you permission to perform surgery and make further decisions during surgery without my consent?"

"Essentially, yes," the doctor confirmed. "You will be under anaesthetic at the time so we can't ask you then, can we?" He raised his eyebrows as he smiled at her. Ariena did not smile back. She put the pen down and sat back in her chair. "I'm not going to sign that, Doctor," she said in a calm, steady voice. "I need to know more about the surgery procedure before I can decide whether there will be any surgery at all," she said, trying to keep her voice steady. "I was led to believe that the recommended surgery would be to remove the tumour only. Under no circumstances whatsoever, will I give you permission to remove my breast without further consultation." Before the doctor could reply, she continued. "I understand fully that my body has been compromised in some way causing the cancer cells to mutate. I am not in denial of that fact. However, I do take offence to the suggestion that I think my body has betrayed me. I do not think that. My body has not betrayed me, if anything, it is I who has betrayed my body," Ariena said. "Obviously, although not realising it at the time, I have put myself in a position that allowed the cancer to grow."

The doctor smiled again. "There's no point in blaming yourself," he said. "Feeling guilty is no better than being in denial," he added. Ariena felt even more affronted by his assumption that she was feeling guilty, but she let it pass and waited in silence for him to continue. "We are aware that there is a tumour that needs to be removed," he said. "Allow me to elaborate. The surgery is straight forward, we locate the tumour and surgically remove it. At the same time, we take extra tissue from the area surrounding the tumour as an added precaution. We are also able to determine whether the cancer has spread to the lymph nodes and will remove all those that may be affected. If the cancer has spread further, then it is standard protocol to remove the entire breast," he explained. He moved forward and put his elbows on the desk, resting his chin in his hands. "I perform this surgery three or four times a week, it's my job," he said. "That's what I do. You do not need to worry about the surgery, I can take care of that for you, you can trust me."

Ariena looked at him, detecting a hint of compassion, but no understanding of her concern. "It's not the surgery itself that I am concerned about Dr Schwartz," she replied, "and I am certainly not questioning your expertise as a surgeon. I know that you are highly qualified to perform surgery when it is necessary, I'm just not sure that in my case it is necessary. I need time to think about this, that is my main concern. I need time to do my own research and decide for myself whether I will have surgery."

The doctor interjected, "Do you not understand that it is imperative to act immediately to arrest the rapid growth?" he said. "Your cancer is highly aggressive and we have to respond in a highly aggressive manner if we are going to achieve any results. Removing the tumour and all affected areas is the first step. You do not have time to think about it, or to research it for yourself. We have done that for you," he added smiling, but with a note of frustration in his voice.

Ariena sighed. She looked at her hands and noticed that they were shaking. She put them in her lap and took a deep breath. "I understand that this is your perception of the situation," she said, "but it is not mine. I believe that time is *all* I have to allow me to make my own decisions, and it is my decision Doctor," she emphasised.

"It is, after all, my breast and my life we're talking about here." The doctor looked somewhat astonished, but said nothing. "I believe there may be merit in removing the tumour in the hope that it may slow down the growth," Ariena said, "but I'm not convinced. Removing the tumour will only slow down the process, it does not address the cause." She was no longer speaking directly to the doctor, she was thinking out loud. "Removing the entire breast would be the same, only much more traumatic to the body, and emotionally to me," she reasoned. "There has to be a more natural way to assist the body to reverse the problem, without invasive surgery or treatment that will compromise it further."

"We're not here to address the cause," the doctor interrupted her train of thought. "The surgery is to slow any further growth, so that we will have the time to give you further treatment that may arrest the cancer. This is the protocol that the medical profession goes by and what we are offering to you."

"The way I see it, Doctor," Ariena said, looking directly at him, "is, if we don't address the cause, it wont matter how much surgery or treatment I have to slow down or arrest the growth, the cancer will eventually return."

"As I said before, I do this surgery three to four times a week. Surgery for breast cancer is increasing in this area. There is a waiting list for all types of surgery. People are having surgery when it becomes necessary so they can get on with their lives. You are lucky in a way that your cancer is highly aggressive," he added. "That has given you priority on the list, but you need to make a decision today, otherwise you may lose that opportunity."

*

Ariena ignored his exasperated manner and replied, "You say that breast cancer is increasing in this area, why is that? Have there been any studies done as to the cause for this increase?"

"I believe there was a study done on the increased pollution from the industries in the area," he replied, "but it was not conclusive."

"So, environmental then," she said. "People are breathing in the pollution which raises their toxic load and compromises the body's system." She was thinking aloud again. The doctor looked at his watch again. "I'm sorry," he said, "I have other patients waiting to see me. We need to conclude this conversation. I can see that you are interested in pursuing this line of thinking. However, I am a surgeon. In your current circumstance I can only offer you surgery. You have an appointment for the day after tomorrow to have the tumour removed. You need to sign this form now, if you wish to keep that surgery appointment."

"Thank you, Doctor," Ariena said, "I appreciate the time you have given me, our conversation has been most enlightening. However, assuming you have told me everything I need to know about the surgery procedure, I'm convinced that I must take the time to do more research before making a decision on whether I will accept your offer of surgery. I will take my chances on getting another appointment if I decide to go ahead."

She stood up and added, "I'm assuming I can telephone your receptionist to advise when I have made my decision?" The doctor appeared somewhat taken aback as he also stood. "Yes," he affirmed, "but don't leave it too long. I'll advise her to make a temporary date for early next week. If she hasn't heard from you by Friday she will call you to confirm."

"Thank you, Doctor," Ariena said again, proffering her hand for him to shake. "I will call by Friday." The doctor nodded and returned to his desk. Ariena noticed that he picked up the pen and opened her file. She thought about what he might have written: '*Difficult patient, in denial.*'

# CHAPTER 8
## SURGERY

"Good morning," Ariena greeted the receptionist cheerfully, "is it possible to speak with the doctor for a few minutes?"

"I'll ask if he will take your call," came the reply. Ariena checked the questions she had listed while she waited.

"Good morning," the doctor's voice brought her back to the phone.

"Good morning, Doctor Schwartz, it's Ariena, I just need to clarify a couple of things before I can make a final decision as to the surgery."

"Yes," he said in a noncommittal tone.

"I've been doing some research as to the timing of surgery to the breast area," she stated. "Apparently, the timing of the surgery and a woman's hormonal cycle may have a positive or negative affect on it's outcome."

"I have never heard of that theory," the doctor replied.

"Well, it does make sense," Ariena suggested, "and the studies show that if the surgery is performed at the correct stage of the hormonal cycle, the affect is more likely to have a positive outcome."

"If I had to time every surgery around the patient's hormonal cycle it would be a nightmare," came the reply, "it would be impossible."

"I'm sure it wouldn't be easy," she acquiesced. "However, if I'm going to have surgery, I want to be sure that everything is taken into account that may help assure a positive outcome. Therefore, I've looked at my dates and if I agree to the surgery, the best timing for me will be in two weeks." The doctor sighed audibly. "If that is when you want the surgery, we can have a look on the schedule to see if there is an opening," he said flatly.

"Right," Ariena said, looking at her notes. "You mentioned the possibility that the cancer may have spread to the lymph nodes and that if so you would remove those affected."

"That is correct. If any are affected, we remove all the lymph nodes present at the time of surgery," he elaborated, "just as we remove some extra tissue around the tumour. That is to ensure that we have got everything we can at the time." He sounded pleased with himself.

"Well," she continued, "my research tells me that removing any lymph nodes compromises the performance of the lymphatic system. As the lymphatic system's job is to remove toxins from the body," she reasoned, "that would not be optimal, since there is every likelihood that the cause of the cancer is due to an overload of toxins." Not waiting for an answer, she went on, "Also, studies have proven that removal of lymph nodes already affected by the cancer, makes no difference to the mortality rate. However, there is a substantial difference to the lymphatic system's effectiveness, as well as the possibility of losing some use of the arm." She paused. "Therefore," Ariena concluded, "*if* I agree to surgery, it will be on the basis that no lymph nodes be removed, irrespective of whether there are any affected or not." There was a brief silence on the phone.

"I see," the doctor said eventually, "well, that is your decision. It's certainly not my recommendation," he added.

"Yes, you are right Doctor, it is my decision," she agreed, "and I think I've already made myself clear that under no circumstance will I agree to having the entire breast removed."

"I have made a note of that," he replied. "but again, it's not my recommendation. A partial or full mastectomy may slow down and even arrest the spread of cancer if performed in time. If it is recommended and you don't agree until a later date, it may be too late," he added.

"I know that is your logic," Ariena said, "but it doesn't make sense to me. How is it that there have been cases of women having had a mastectomy, or even both breasts removed," she emphasised, "and the cancer has appeared elsewhere later?"

"It is relatively common that breast cancer can spread to other areas of the body, particularly the bones," he replied. "Once in the bones there is little that can be done, that is why it is crucial to do everything we can before it spreads any further."

"Then clearly, removal of the breast is a gamble, just as removal of the tumour is. It's just another way to slow things down – *maybe*," she added. "To be honest, Doctor," she continued, "I will not agree to having my breast removed now or later, regardless of any recommendations or possible outcomes. They are my breasts and I'll be taking them with me, whether sooner, or later," Ariena proclaimed. She took a deep breath and continued, "I accept that surgery to remove the tumour *may* slow things down, if it hasn't already spread further. That is the only reason I would agree to having surgery at all. It may give me time to identify and eliminate the cause, which is clearly what really needs to be done."

"So, are you saying that you want the surgery, or not?" the doctor asked. Ariena let the moment of indecision pass. She nodded to herself. "I will agree to having surgery only to remove the tumour, but it must be at the correct time of my cycle," she said. "If there is no available opening then I will wait another month."

"We have you booked in for next week, waiting another month may be waiting too long," the doctor warned again.

"That is a gamble I'm willing to take, Doctor," she replied.

*

The hospital gown fell open at the back as Ariena bent over to put the paper slippers on her feet. She straightened up and tried to reach the ties on the back of the gown. *You have to be a contortionist to get it done up*, she thought. She reached lower, but there were no other ties. *I don't get it*, she thought. *Why does the opening have to be at the back? It's ridiculous, especially as it's breast surgery! God, I hope they know the breasts are at the front!* She chuckled at the humour of her situation. Grabbing a handful of gown in her hand and holding it together at the back, she walked out of the changing room, tucking the gown under herself as she sat down in the waiting room. She raised her eyebrows at the other people also in hospital gowns, sitting equally as awkwardly on their chairs. "Not exactly elegant, are they?" she said with a comical grimace.

"I can never figure out why they have to be done up at the back," a young woman replied.

"Why they *don't* do up at the back, more like," an older woman remarked.

"It's a joke," an elderly gentleman said. "What else is there to laugh about around here?"

Ariena smiled. "Well, I guess you have to see the funny side of it," she replied.

"Yep," he agreed with a grin. "See some pretty funny *back* sides!" Hearing her name called, Ariena stood, and holding her gown together at the back, took a step forward.

"Hold onto it girl," the elderly gentleman smiled at her, "don't let go of what's yours." Although she smiled at his further attempt to lighten the situation with humour, she couldn't help thinking how ominous his words were.

*

With rising apprehension, she followed the nurse down the corridor and into the lift. The nurse said nothing as the lift rose and stopped at the next floor. The doors opened and she stepped out, waiting for Ariena to follow.

"There must be some mistake," Ariena said, looking at the sign above the door, "this is Maternity."

"Yes, that's right," the nurse agreed, "you wait here to be called to surgery."

"But I'm not having a baby," Ariena replied anxiously.

The nurse laughed. "Well, that is obvious, love. No, we're using the maternity visitor's room for holding before women's surgery," she explained.

"That could be a little confusing for the visitors," Ariena commented with relief.

"Don't worry love, you just wait here and I'll come and get you when they're ready for you." Ariena sat down, tucking her gown beneath her again. She was trying to see the funny side of this situation, but her sense of humour was rapidly diminishing.

She smiled at the other patients seated in their gowns, none of them looked pregnant and all appeared unperturbed by their surroundings. She picked up a magazine and flipped through it absently, trying to convince herself that all was normal and that there was nothing to be concerned about. But the nagging apprehension would not go away. She stood up and looked out the window. The view gave her no solace. The dark red water stains on the stark grey concrete wall looked like congealed blood, another scene from a horror movie. She turned away from the window and started to walk along the corridor towards the nursery. Perhaps if she could see the newborn babies in their cribs she would feel better. Ariena felt the warmth of love flood over her as she gazed at their tiny faces, with no sign of apprehension as they slept soundly in their little cribs.

"They're so angelic when they are asleep," the nurse commented as she approached.

"Yes, almost makes you want to start over," Ariena said with a smile.

"Well, you wont be doing that after today's surgery," the nurse replied. Ariena turned and looked at her. "What do you mean?" she asked, somewhat bewildered by the nurse's comment.

"Well, you wont be getting pregnant after having a hysterectomy, lovey," she replied.

"A what?"

"Says here you're in for a hysterectomy," the nurse flipped open the chart she was holding. Ariena stared at her in shocked disbelief. "No, no, there's definitely a mistake here. I'm not in for a hysterectomy, although that would be preferable," she added, "I'm in for a breast lumpectomy."

"Oh, goodness," the nurse gasped, "are you sure?"

"Are you kidding?" countered Ariena.

"We'd better go to the desk and sort this out before they call you in."

"You're not kidding, are you?" Ariena couldn't believe what she was hearing. The lift doors opened and several people stepped out, amongst them a woman Ariena knew.

"Hello," the woman said cheerfully, "in for surgery? Mine's hysterectomy, how about you?"

"I hate to tell you this," Ariena replied, "but you're too late, I'm having the hysterectomy. It's OK though, you can have a mastectomy instead, I'm happy to swap!"

"You what?"

"Sorry, couldn't resist," Ariena said with a laugh, "you have to keep you sense of humour around here, otherwise you'll lose it completely! I've just been told that I'm in for a hysterectomy, but

I'm actually here for breast surgery, supposedly to remove a lump, *not* the whole breast."

"You'd better come with us to sort this out," the nurse interrupted.

"Well, you're right there," Ariena said, winking at her friend.

*

The nurse handed Ariena a paper cap that looked like a shower cap. "Pop this on to complete your outfit love," she said. "Down the corridor and go through the third door on the right," she instructed. "Straight ahead and there's another waiting area at the end. Wait there for the prep nurse, OK?"

As she went through the third door, it clicked shut behind her. Looking back at it, she realised it was a one-way door. *That's it then, no going back.* The humour left her as she walked towards the end of the hallway, her paper slippers making a shuffling sound on the polished tiled floor. She looked ahead at the large double doors with 'NO ENTRY' printed in bold red across the middle. There was no-one to be seen. She stopped at the double doors. To the left, a small area was portioned off with a counter in front. She looked behind the counter at the empty chair. There was nothing on the desk. She turned around and looked back up the hallway and saw a small alcove, a single bed on wheels parked against the wall. She walked over to the bed and gave it a push, it didn't move. She leaned up against the bed and surveyed the scene again. The walls and ceiling were stark white. The tiled floor, white with tiny flecks, was so highly polished she could see her reflection in it. Apart from the bed and the chair behind the counter, there was no other furniture. No sign of a waiting room and no sound other than her breathing.

*

A feeling of foreboding swept over her as she thought. *I must be in the wrong place.* She knew there was no point in trying the door she had come through, there was nothing to open it from this side. She had assumed the double doors led to an operating theatre, but began to wonder. *What if I am in the wrong place and that's not a theatre? It might just lead outside. Or to another realm,* she thought with an attempt at amusing herself. She hoisted herself onto the edge of the bed and sat there, staring at the NO ENTRY sign on the doors. *Wonder what would happen if I was to open those doors?* She imagined there being an operating table surrounded by doctors, with bright spotlights shining down on an inert body on the table. She imagined the flurry of nurses rushing to stop her from entering the room. "Hello?" she called out. No answer. No sound. *OK, this is seriously weird,* she thought. *Maybe I'm not meant to be here, at all. Maybe I should never have agreed to the surgery.* The foreboding feeling began to surround her. She started walking towards the door she had come through. *Maybe someone will hear me if I bang on the door.* The closer she got to the shut door, the more anxious she became. She reached the door and stopped. She could feel her heart thumping in her chest. *I've got to get out,* she thought and making a fist, she reached towards the door.

"Ariena? What are you doing? You should be resting on the bed," a voice behind her made her jump. She turned to see a nurse walking towards her, a door standing open beyond the counter behind her.

"I didn't see that door," Ariena blurted out. "I thought I was in the wrong place."

"Not if you're here for surgery," the nurse replied brightly. "This is the right place. Come along, let's get you prepped, the anaesthetist will be here shortly to see you."

"Is it too late to change my mind?" Ariena heard the plaintive question slip out. The nurse didn't appear to hear her.

*

After telling Ariena to lie on the bed and relax, the nurse had left her alone again. Ariena tried to calm herself by meditating. She sat up, assuming the yoga lotus position and closed her eyes. Slowly she breathed deeply and cleared her mind. When the anaesthetist arrived she was feeling much more in control of herself and resigned to her decision to go ahead with the surgery. She answered all the questions that the anaesthetist asked that confirmed she was the patient on the chart.

"I have a couple of questions for you," Ariena said. "Now that we've ascertained that I am me," she smiled, "can you please confirm what surgery I am to have? It's just that the nurse in the ward thought I was in for something different, so I'd like to know before I have the anaesthetic that I'm having the right surgery."

"That's a good question to ask. According to this chart, your surgery is for a lumpectomy, removal of a tumour in the left breast," the anaesthetist replied.

"Yes, that's correct," Ariena said with relief, but feeling odd at the irony that she would be relieved to be having surgery at all. "Something else you wanted to ask?"

"Yes, about the anaesthetic."

"Ah, yes, I was getting to that. The anaesthetic consists of three different drugs, one to put you to sleep, the other two are for the pain, so that as you regain consciousness, the pain is minimal," she explained. "Once you are fully conscious, you can have the option of taking tablets or we can set up a drip for self-administered pain relief if you prefer."

"Well, I would prefer to have no pain relief drugs at all. I don't even take aspirin for pain, let alone anything stronger," Ariena replied.

"You will need pain relief for the surgery," the anaesthetist assured her. "It is always added to the anaesthetic. Once it wears off, you can gauge the pain and take relief as you wish."

"I've had surgery before and I experienced severe nausea afterwards. I was told that it is the anaesthetic that causes the nausea," Ariena said.

"It's the morphine that causes the nausea," she explained.

"Oh no, I really don't want morphine at all," Ariena persisted. "Is it absolutely necessary? What is the other pain killer?"

"Demerol, and it's not usually sufficient on it's own. The morphine dose could be lowered if you insist," came the reply. "However, as the anaesthetist I am responsible for the patient's welfare during surgery, so I must advise you that I will take whatever precautions or action that is required if I deem it necessary."

"I understand that, thank you," Ariena said, "but you will initially lower the dose of morphine?"

"Yes, I can do that," she replied with a smile. "Don't worry, we'll take good care of you."

"Thank you," Ariena repeated, "I trust you will."

"You lie down and relax now," the anaesthetist said patting her arm, "I'll be back for you in about 15 minutes and we'll be going in."

*

*Why did I agree to this?* Ariena agonised to herself. She lay down and closed her eyes. She didn't want to see this space anymore. She didn't want to be left alone in it again. She opened her eyes and looked over at the NO ENTRY sign. In her mind she imagined a beautiful scene behind the doors, with trees and flowers and birds and butterflies, and she thought of herself walking through into another realm, a place with no doubts, no fear, no cancer.

She felt the sting of the needle going into her arm and sensed the fluid entering her vein. She closed her eyes against the glare of the lights. A sickly sweet metallic taste crept into the back of her throat.

"I can taste it," she said without opening her eyes.

"That's OK, love," someone said, "wont be for long."

"I want you to count down from 10 for me," she heard the anaesthetist say.

She thought, *Count down, that's weird.*

"You can start now, 10," the voice prompted her.

"OK," she slowly started counting, "10, nine, eight, seven, six." She stopped, there was a moment's silence.

"She's under," someone said.

"No, I'm not," Ariena contradicted the voice, "I was just thinking; *what if I get to zero*?"

"Keep counting love, you got to six."

"Five," she said. "Fourrrr," she heard her own voice trailing into the distance. "Thrrrr," her voice disappeared as she felt herself drifting, drifting, drifting. There was no beautiful realm with flowers and birds and butterflies, only darkness.

\*

"Hello, welcome back to the land of the living." Ariena heard her friend's voice and felt a warm hand on her own. She opened her eyes. "We've got to stop meeting like this, Doctor," she said, smiling at her friend.

"I agree," Dr Dubois replied, "I much prefer meeting in the garden or the sauna."

"Yes, let's do that this week," Ariena said.

"Which? The garden or the sauna?"

"Both of course," Ariena laughed.

"Ah, good, sounds like you are back to your usual self. That was quick, must have been the reiki," she said with a wink.

"Yes, I feel relatively normal, thanks," Ariena said with a smile, "and no nausea, they must have lowered the morphine dose."

"I heard about that," the doctor said, checking her pulse, "good call," she added. "How is the pain?"

"Can't feel anything," Ariena replied, suddenly putting her hand on the bandaged breast.

"It's OK," her friend reassured her, "she's still there."

"Whew!" Ariena lay back on the pillow and closed her eyes momentarily.

"You might as well have another snooze," the doctor said, "just to sleep it off. I'll come back and see you in an hour, when you'll feel more like talking."

"Mmm, OK," Ariena didn't open her eyes. She slept soundly for three hours, not waking when Dr Dubois returned, not feeling her bed being wheeled to the ward, not hearing the clatter of meal trays come and go in her room.

"She's still asleep," the nurse was saying, "do you think I should hook up the pain relief for when she comes around?"

"Probably a good idea," another nurse said, "that may wake her anyway."

"I am awake," Ariena said, opening her eyes, "and I don't need any pain relief, thank you."

"Ah, there you are," said the nurse, "are you sure about the pain relief?"

"Yes, I'm sure," Ariena said.

"It may not have fully worn off yet," the nurse said, "I can hook you up so you can self administer, or I can give you tablets if you prefer."

"Please, just leave the tablets," Ariena didn't want to argue. "Did my doctor come?"

"Yes, dear," the nurse put the tablets on her table and poured a glass of water. "She didn't want to wake you so she's put you in here overnight. She'll be around in the morning after breakfast." Ariena sat up and reached for the water. "Now if you need us for anything," the nurse said, "you just push this little button. Don't go putting up with any pain, you can have more tablets in a couple of hours if you need them."

"Thank you. I'm just really thirsty right now, can I have a jug of water," Ariena asked.

"Of course you can," the nurse filled a jug and put it on her bedside table. "Anything else?"

"No, thank you," she replied, pouring another glass of water.

"Don't forget to take the tablets with that," the nurse said, smiling as she left the room. Ariena reached for the tablets, opened the drawer in the bedside table and placed the little paper cup with the tablets inside the drawer. She closed the drawer. "End of discussion," she whispered, and drank the rest of the water.

*

As she suspected, breakfast was inedible. "Are you not hungry?" the nurse asked, clearing the tray. "Do you feel all right, love?"

"I'm fine, thank you," Ariena replied. "I don't eat bacon and eggs, toast or coffee. Is there any fresh fruit available?"

"Really?" the nurse looked perplexed, "Fresh fruit? I don't think so dear, maybe at lunch. Would you like to order it?"

"That's OK," Ariena said, "it was just a question really. I'm sure I wont be here for lunch."

A different nurse arrived with a little paper cup and put it on her table. "Your tablets, for the pain," she explained, seeing the questioning look on Ariena's face.

"Thank you, but I don't need them," she said.

"Oh, they're on your chart dear," the nurse said, "you have to have them." Ariena sighed. She picked up the little cup and poured a glass of water. The nurse satisfied, moved on to the next bed. Ariena opened the drawer and placed the cup inside, then quietly closed the drawer. *I suppose people are usually so drugged up, they wouldn't know whether they need pain relief or not*, she thought. She tentatively put her hand on her bandaged breast and gently applied some pressure. Yep, there it is, pain! *Not so you need drugs for it though*, she thought.

*

"Hey, you," Dr Dubois called approaching her bed. "You sure had a good sleep, I couldn't wake you when I came back last night."

"You didn't try," Ariena suggested with a smile.

"You're right," her friend said with a laugh as she pulled the curtains around her bed.

"Yay, privacy," Ariena said with a chuckle. "Before I forget, there's some pain killers lurking in the drawer here." She reached over and opened the drawer. "Don't want the next unsuspecting patient to find them. Here you go, Doctor," she put the tablets in her friend's hand, "you can take care of them."

"You brat," she said, putting them in her pocket.

"Well, Doc," Ariena said jovially, "what's the verdict?"

"Let's take a look at you," the doctor said, ignoring her question. Ariena watched as she undid the bandage. She breathed a sigh of relief to see her breast still there.

"I can't see the incision, how does it look?" she asked.

"Very neat and tidy," the doctor replied, carefully replacing the bandage. "Still minimal pain?"

"Yep, only when I breathe," Ariena replied jokingly, "but, you didn't answer my question."

"Well, what would you like first, the good news or the bad?"

"I already saw the good news," Ariena said smiling at her breast, "might as well hit me with the bad."

"It's no joke, my friend," the doctor said with a solemn look, "it *is* bad news, I'm afraid."

"Well, here's the deal," Ariena replied, "I've already decided that there will be no fear involved in this, whatever the outcome," she said. "It's a negative emotion and there's no place for it in my life. Fear only causes irrational behaviour that may be dangerous, especially when making what may be life dependent decisions." She looked squarely at her friend. "So, don't you be afraid either," she said smiling. "Tell me the way it is, I can handle it, honestly," she assured her, "and don't start with 'I'm sorry' just give me the facts." Her friend sat on the edge of the bed and looked in her eyes. "OK, I'm glad to hear it," she said, "you're going to need all the courage you can muster for this one." She took a deep breath before she continued. "The tumour was about the size of a golf ball. They removed it along with a substantial amount of surrounding tissue, so about the size of an orange all told was taken from behind the breast. There were also nine out of 23 lymph nodes present that were affected. They were able to remove all the nodes present without having to make a second incision…"

"What?" Ariena interrupted, "I specifically said I did not want any lymph nodes removed."

"I know, but I believe the decision was made to try to arrest further growth," the doctor replied.

"The surgeon agreed not to remove the lymph nodes," Ariena insisted.

"I'm…" her friend stopped herself saying sorry, "they removed all 23 present," she said flatly.

Ariena took a deep breath. "I also refuse to engage in anger," she stated, "another negative emotion that will do no good. However, I *will* be speaking to the surgeon about trust," she added. She looked back at her friend and smiled. "You mentioned further growth?" she prompted.

"Yes, there was no other growth visible within the breast tissue, but there is some present in the chest wall," her doctor continued, "there are numerous smaller tumours scattered throughout the chest wall, too many and over too wide an area to remove. The rapid spread of the cancer is evident, as was suspected." She dropped her gaze but not before Ariena detected a look of sadness in her eyes. "That's why they took the lymph nodes," she concluded.

"We both know that wont make any difference," Ariena said, "not to the rate of growth."

"They will recommend chemotherapy and radiation to try to get the rest," the doctor said.

"Brilliant," Ariena muttered. She adjusted the pillow behind her and leaned back. "You know that's not an option for me," she stated.

"It may be possible to tolerate it with complimentary therapy," her doctor suggested.

"What do you mean?"

"I think you should get the recommendations from the oncologist and then go see our friend the naturopathic physician," she replied, "rather than refuse the treatment outright," she added. "He may have several options that you could consider."

"Yes, of course, you're right," Ariena said, "I will do that. Do I have an appointment to see the oncologist already?"

"Yes, and a follow up with the surgeon," she added raising her eyebrows. "Don't be too hard on him, as with all of us, he has a responsibility to his patient to do the best he can."

\*

Ariena had been at home a week when she awoke one morning with a strange sensation in her chest. The pain from her surgery had abated with each day and the incision was healing rapidly. So, as she rolled over readying herself to sit up and get out of bed, the unusual sensation she experience shocked her. "What was that?" she said to herself as she put her hand to her breast. She looked down at her breast, but couldn't see anything unusual. She cupped the breast and gently lifted it, immediately feeling the odd sensation again. It was not like the pain she'd been feeling since the surgery, not even a bruised feeling, but rather a pulling, stinging sensation.

A wave of dread washed over her, this sensation did not feel right. She carefully sat up and slowly swung her legs over the side of the bed. She felt like the sensation was lurking in the background, and that her movements would trigger it again.

She slowly rose and took a tentative step towards the mirror, carefully following with another step until she stood directly in front of it. She had not looked at herself in the mirror for weeks, her busy days being taken up with research or appointments, getting dressed in the mornings had been a rushed affair. As she looked at her naked body, she forgot for a moment why she was there. She appraised how shapely her body looked and thought briefly that it wasn't bad for a woman in her fifties. Then her eyes lit on her breasts and she noticed for the first time that they were no longer equal in size or shape. The incision glared at her, a dark gash down the side of her breast, crusty with a forming scab. A deep hollow beneath the gash, where the tumour and surrounding tissue had been removed had sunken at the side of her breast, causing the nipple to point directly forward instead of slightly downwards as it had done before. She thought how ironic it was that the surgery had reduced the breast in size, which had given it a perky look. The other breast looked the same as before, it's fullness hanging slightly on her ribcage. She thought perhaps if she raised her arms above her head they would even out, so she did, and immediately wished she hadn't.

"Ow," she exclaimed, as she felt the sensation again, this time intermingled with a sharp pain. She felt again the wave of foreboding, something was wrong. Slowly, very carefully, she raised her arms again. This time it felt more like a tearing sensation, deep inside her breast. She continued to slowly raise her arm fully, then cupping her breast gently with her other hand, she slowly lifted it.

"Oh my God!" she gasped, as she stared at the underside of her breast. Deep purple streaks and red blotches showed through the tissue appearing like bruising, but the colour was wrong. She continued to stare, shocked at what she saw and for a moment, forgot about the strange sensation she had felt. Dropping her arm by her side, the tearing sensation ripped through her breast and into her chest, making her cry out in shock and pain. She took a step back and sat down on the bed, not taking her hand from her breast. She could feel her heart beating against her chest and hear it thudding in her ears. Tears sprang to her eyes and she let out a sob involuntarily. She faltered in her breathing, and took a few gasps of air, realising that she really was in shock. She stood up again, keeping in mind to move slowly, and reached for her robe that was hanging on the door. She carefully put first one arm then the other into the robe and pulled it around her, then grasping the door handle to steady herself, she staggered through into the hallway, feeling like she was moving in slow motion. She reached the telephone and, picking up the handset, she dialled her doctor's number.

\*

"Good thing you phoned when you did," Dr Dubois said, "I was just about to leave for the clinic. I'll call in on my way, should be there in about 10 minutes. Meanwhile, make yourself a cup of tea and relax, it's probably nothing to be too concerned about."

"Thanks," Ariena replied, "I hope you're right." She went into the kitchen and put the kettle on, then returned to her bedroom to get dressed, trying to contain her fear that something was terribly wrong.

"You're such a good friend," Ariena said, letting the doctor in. "Thanks for calling in, you could have told me to make an appointment at the clinic."

"I was literally driving past your door, best to call in and quell your fears," her friend replied, "so, let's take a look at what you've got there." They went into the bedroom and Ariena sat down and opened her shirt.

"There's something not right about the discolouration," Ariena commented, "it doesn't look like bruising, and it didn't appear until now, usually you see bruising sooner. This almost looks like internal bleeding to me." The doctor gently applied pressure to the breast as she examined the area that was so vividly discoloured.

"Hmm," she murmured, and placing her hand on the breast she said, "lift your arm up slowly." Ariena winced as she complied. "It's odd, it's painful, but more like a tearing sensation," she said. The doctor lowered Ariena's arm gently and smiled at her. "Well, it's as I thought," she said, "and your description is fairly accurate. The tearing sensation you are feeling is exactly that. As you move, or more precisely, as you stretch the surgical area, the tissue that is in the process of healing, is tearing apart again."

"It's tearing?" Ariena questioned, "Really? Why would it be tearing? It's not like I'm doing anything extreme."

"The tissue is not tearing apart from itself," the doctor corrected her, "it's tearing away from the staples. The discolouration you can see is minute bleeding from the hairline tears, but you don't need to worry about it, it's a normal response. You just need to be careful with your movements for the next week or so to allow it to fuse enough so that it will not tear away. We could bind the area and your arm if that will help." Ariena had stopped buttoning her shirt and was staring at her friend. "Did you say, *staples*?" she asked. "What staples, what are you talking about?"

"The surgeon didn't tell you?"

"Didn't tell me what?"

"OK," Dr Dubois put her hand on Ariena's arm, "once the surgery is complete, staples are used to hold the tissue together while it is healing. It's normal procedure these days, so that's probably why the surgeon didn't mention it." Ariena shook her head as if to clear her mind. "Hold on, let me get this straight," she said, "you're telling me that the surgeon doesn't sew you up anymore, that he uses *staples*? What kind of staples, and how does he use them?" The doctor patted her arm. "Don't fret," she said, smiling at her friend, "it's nothing to get upset about. Yes, staples are used instead of literally sewing you up, the staples are surgical steel, completely safe and hygienic, and they use a device similar to a staple gun. It's very quick and enables the tissue to heal just as well as with using dissolving stitches." Ariena sat with a dumbfounded look on her face. "I don't believe it," she eventually said, shaking her head. "So, now I have steel staples in my breast? No wonder the tissue is having a hard time healing, how is it supposed to adhere to steel? No wonder it's tearing apart!"

"Ari, it's OK," the doctor said, continuing to pat her arm.

"Given time, the tissue will heal around and over the staples, they are there to hold things together while the healing takes place, like the stitches did when they were used. You have to be patient and aware of your movements for a couple more weeks and it will be fine." Ariena finished buttoning her shirt and stood up, looking aghast at her friend. "No Fran," she said with a steady voice, "no, it's not OK. It's not OK to shoot my already compromised breast full of steel staples that are not going to dissolve. It's not OK for a skilled surgeon to use a staple gun instead of sewing the tissue in place, and no, it's not OK that the surgeon did not mention this so-called procedure beforehand!"

"Oh, Ari," her friend said, "I'm so sorry that you were not made aware of that part of the procedure, but to be honest, everything is just part of the overall procedure. There are so many procedures that are used during surgery that surgeons could not advise the patient of them all."

"I specifically asked him if there was anything to do with the procedure during surgery that I should know about," Ariena replied defiantly, "and furthermore, if I'd known he was going to use staples, maybe I should have been talking to a skilled carpenter!" The doctor smiled. "I know you are not joking," she said, "but that remark was kind of humorous. If it makes you feel any better about the surgeon, it's not actually him who puts the staples in."

"Oh? So who does it then?" She looked at Ariena and smiled again. "I think they call in a skilled carpenter." Ariena couldn't help smiling. "This really is not a laughing matter," she said, "how is this going to affect my physical exercise? Am I going to have tearing of the tissue every time I move?"

"This procedure has been used for some time now, it's considered normal practice, so try not to be upset over it," Dr Dubois replied, "you'll be fine once everything is healed. It is considered however, that breast cancer patients who have had surgery, should be more careful about their upper body movements and should not participate in extreme exercise."

"Oh, great," Ariena said. "So I'm to be an invalid now?"

"No, of course not," her friend replied, "might want to stay off the tennis court though."

\*

While Ariena waited for the scheduled follow-up appointment with the surgeon, she spent the interim doing further research on the consensus of physical activity after breast cancer surgery. Most of the information through medical resources was vague, although there were a few references to the theory that upper body exercise should be kept to a minimum, especially if the patient had any lymph nodes removed. However, she was encouraged to discover a recent research project that had been conducted by a sports medicine physician. The physician believed that upper body exercise had a role in recovery from breast cancer and lymphoaedema because it could improve the range of motion and reverse muscle atrophy, it could also activate skeletal muscle which might help pump lymph and stimulate the immune system. The study looked at the cardio-respiratory fitness levels in two groups of women; one group had been treated for breast cancer, and the other group had no history of breast cancer. The breast cancer group had many anecdotal stories about the 'don'ts' they had been told after treatment. Most of this advice restricted activities involving the upper body. Though well intentioned, there was no published research that supported this information. A desire to return these individuals to an unrestricted, active lifestyle, as well as the lack of scientific proof to the contrary, was the impetus behind the idea to form the first all breast cancer survivors' dragon boat team. The only criteria to join the team was a history of breast cancer. Age, athletic ability, paddling experience were not considered. Dragon boating was chosen for several reasons. It is a strenuous, repetitive upper body activity. It uses predominantly upper extremity and trunk muscles, and the improvement in strength has a carry-over effect to day-to-day activity. The findings were compelling. The paddlers showed a marked improvement in both physical and mental health and there were no cases of lymphoaedema. Ariena decided she would join a dragon boat team herself, it was a positive step that made her feel like she was taking control of her life.

*

Ariena walked into the surgeon's office with purpose to her step.

"Hello," Dr Schwartz greeted her cheerfully, "how are you feeling now?"

"Very annoyed," Ariena replied as she sat down.

"Oh?" he said, looking a little rebuked, "and why is that?"

"*That*, is because you did not tell me everything about the surgery procedure beforehand, even though I specifically asked you," she replied, and before he could answer she continued, "why did you not mention that you would be using staples instead of sewing the tissue together after the surgery?"

"Oh, *that*," he said, looking more relieved, "we haven't used the old catgut method for years."

"*That* does not answer my question," Ariena said, looking at the surgeon steadily.

"It's just normal procedure these days," he explained, "it's not something we even *think* to mention to the patient. Are you having any post-surgery trauma to the site?" he asked, dismissing the previous topic.

"The only trauma I've experienced was first, feeling the tearing sensation in my breast, second, discovering the alarming discolouration to the tissue and not knowing what was causing either, and third, being informed that it was all due to having *staples* permanently lodged in my breast!" she replied with indignation.

"Dr Dubois explained it to you then," he said, "that's good, so you understand that there is nothing to be concerned about, just take it easy for the next couple of weeks while it heals, then be aware that you should avoid strenuous exercise in the future." Dr Schwatz opened a file on his desk and picking up a pen, starting making notes in the file as if the discussion was closed.

"Quote, unquote," Ariena muttered under her breath. The surgeon looked up. "What was that?" he asked.

"Oh, nothing," Ariena said with a sigh.

"Right, so everything is fine then," he stated, rather than asked.

"No, not exactly," she contradicted him. "Dr Dubois also informed me that you removed all the lymph nodes present, *including* those that were not affected," Ariena said accusingly.

"Yes, that is correct," the surgeon replied. "Considering the amount affected and the spread of cancer into the chest wall, I deemed it prudent to do so," he explained.

"Despite the fact that removing the lymph nodes has no affect on the mortality rate," Ariena said, "and, *you* agreed *not* to remove any lymph nodes whatever the outcome," she reminded him.

"I did warn you that I would make that decision during surgery, depending on what we found," he said with finality.

"We discussed and agreed that the decision was mine to make," Ariena insisted. "You also told me that I could trust you. Well, I have to say, that trust has been broken." She looked directly at him and asked, "Is there anything else you have *not* told me regarding the surgery procedures, Doctor?" He avoided her gaze and looked at the file on his desk again. "I don't think so, we've covered everything," he said without looking up, "your appointment at the Cancer Clinic to see the oncologist is for Friday," he passed her an appointment note. "When you get under way with the recommended treatment, we can talk again about the possibility of a mastectomy." Ariena stared at him incredulously. "What did you say?" she asked, knowing exactly what he had said.

"If the treatment goes well," Dr Schwartz began to explain, "that is, if there is a reduction of growth in the chest wall due to the treatment, then there will be no need to remove the breast, since it does not appear to be affected now that the tumour is removed," he continued. "However, if there is no improvement, then we must assume that we did not get all the cancer from the breast area during surgery. Then a mastectomy would be necessary to be absolutely sure." Ariena remained silent, but the surgeon did not elaborate further. He was busy putting the papers into her file, as if the matter was closed. Ariena stood up. "Is that all?" she asked him.

"Yes," he said looking up and smiling, "for the moment."

"Well, thank you Doctor," she said. "There *is* one thing you can be absolutely sure about," she added as she took a step towards the door, "and that is, when I walk through that door, you will not be seeing me again." Dr Schwartz stood up and was about to say something when Ariena cut him short. "I can assure you that I *will* beat this cancer," she said with confidence, "but any further decisions to be made will be *mine*," she added with defiance. "Good day to you Doctor." She opened the door and without looking back, she continued through the outside doors and onto the street. *I'm sure I will not be remembered as a saint around here, she thought to herself, I'm certainly no Saint Catherine or Saint Agatha. They complied, but I wont have my breasts cut off for anyone!*

# CHAPTER 9
# THE TREATMENT

"I am so glad you came," Ariena said to Scott as they drove together to the Cancer Clinic.

"That's what family's all about Mum," he replied smiling at her. "How's it been going with the research?"

"Hectic. There's so much to find out and it's been hard to find the time with having tests and the surgery," she replied. "Everything seems so rushed. I feel like I'm being forced into making decisions before I have all the facts," she added.

"I know you weren't too happy about having the surgery," he said. "How do you feel about it now?"

"Honestly? From what I've learnt since, I don't think I should have agreed to it."

"Really? Why?" he asked.

"Well, I already knew that surgery does not address the cause of the problem," she replied, "and from what I've been reading recently, there are alternatives to surgery for stopping the growth. There are natural therapies that will shrink the tumour to nothing," she added. "Well, at least having the tumour removed has given you more time to make decisions on the treatment," he said. "We can keep up the research so we find the best solution for whatever presents itself in the future."

"Yes," she agreed, "now we've got the team working on it," she laughed, referring to her daughter Joy and Scott's fiancee Mia. "The girls are finding out all kinds of information that we would otherwise never have known. Seems like the doctors don't have any information on anything other than what the medical profession offers."

"Yes, well, that's not surprising," he said, "when you think about it, it's not in their best interest, is it?"

"I always thought they were supposed to have the patient's best interest at heart."

"Maybe in the old days of family doctors who made house-calls with their little bag of tricks," Scott mused. "That's only on TV series nowadays."

"Well, I know a doctor who has one of those little bag of tricks," Ariena said smiling. "I just might have to give him a call."

"Yes, that's our next project," he agreed. "After we get the information today, we can go see him and compare notes."

"We've got a lot of questions to be answered today, and that's just what we have listed," she said, "I'm sure we'll have more when we hear what they have to say."

*

The waiting room was filled with people. "Wow, there's a few people here," Scott whispered to Ariena, "it's worse than emergency at the hospital."

"That tells you something, doesn't it," she whispered back. He nodded.

The receptionist came into the room and called a name, looking around for the patient. A young woman stood and followed the receptionist down a hallway lined with doors. The receptionist ushered the woman into one of the rooms and closed the door.

"I've been in this scene before," Ariena whispered to her son. "Thank goodness you're with me this time." He reached over and held her hand. "I'll stick with you like glue," he whispered smiling.

"I'm not making any decisions or signing anything today," she said under her breath.

"No way," he agreed, winking at her. "I'm with you on that."

They watched as patient after patient were ushered into various rooms, each of them reappearing back at the reception desk a relatively short time later.

"Do you think they are actually seeing anyone?" Ariena whispered.

"They don't seem to be away very long." Scott shrugged. "Maybe they don't have as many questions as we do," he whispered.

When the reception called her name, they stood up together preparing to follow her.

"You can wait here," the receptionist said to Scott, "she wont be long, about 15 minutes."

"Yes, I've noticed that," he replied, "however, I'll be staying with my mother, thank you." The receptionist appeared surprised. "OK," she said, "follow me then." They smiled at each other as she closed the door. Ariena looked around the room. It was small and appeared cluttered with just the one bed and two chairs. There were no shelves or anything decorating the yellow painted walls.

"Good. No jars," she said as she sat on the side of the bed. Scott laughed, remembering Ariena's story of her visit to the surgeon. He was about to sit down on one of the chairs when a young woman entered the room. She stopped when she saw them both, then glanced at the name on the file she was carrying. She looked slightly confused. Ariena stepped forward and introduced herself and Scott. "My doctor suggested I bring someone with me," she explained. The young woman nodded. "Very good," she said. "I'm Dr Price. Your case has been discussed by the team of oncologists here at the Clinic and I have been appointed as your personal oncologist. Today, I will explain about the treatment that we have decided will be best for you."

Ariena sat back on the edge of the bed.

"You may have this chair," the oncologist offered, "we wont be doing any examination."

"Thank you," Ariena smiled, "I'm fine here, you go ahead." Dr Price remained standing. "According to your pathologist's report," she continued, "you have a highly aggressive form of breast cancer. Your surgeon's report shows that the tumour in the left breast has been removed, along with a substantial amount of surrounding tissue." She glanced at the report in her hand. "There were also nine out of 23 lymph nodes present at the time of surgery that were affected and have also been removed," she read.

"Yes, I'm not happy about that," Ariena interjected. "I specifically asked the surgeon not to remove any lymph nodes." The oncologist held her hand up, ignoring Ariena's comment, and continued, "The surgeon's report indicates that there was no further growth within the breast tissue, but that it was evident within the chest wall. A mastectomy was not performed." Ariena was about to make another comment but thought better of it. "We have considered this report and it is our recommendation that you undergo a course of chemotherapy as well as radiation treatment to the area."

"I have a question," Scott interjected.

"No questions until after I've finished," Dr Price said, looking at him sternly.

"It has to do with what you're talking about now," he countered.

"When I'm finished, there may be time for one or two questions, so please don't interrupt," she said glaring at him.

"OK," he said, shaking his head in disbelief.

*

The oncologist referred to the file and started describing the various types of chemotherapy. As she continued speaking in a monotone, Ariena stopped listening to the details. The young woman's voice sounded like a recording, there were no inflections or emphasis placed on any words, just a monotonous drone that Ariena turned off from her mind. She looked at her son, studiously taking notes, his eyes fixed to his notebook, no longer attempting to enter into a conversation. She wondered if the young woman delivering the oratory realised that she had lost her audience. She looked back at her, there was nothing to indicate that the woman in front of her had any interest in who she was, or what she felt. *This woman has been programmed*, she thought. *Programmed to say what she has to and no more.*

"Of the two that I've just described," Dr Price was saying, "we suggest that the stronger chemotherapy would be best in your case. Your doctor's notes describe you as a physically fit and otherwise healthy individual, therefore you would be able to withstand the stronger side affects of this particular drug."

"What are the side affects?" Ariena heard her son interrupt. She snapped back to join in. "Yes, how strong is this drug?" she asked. The oncologist handed her a sheet of paper. "All the details are on here," she said. "The reason we don't often recommend this one is because the strength of it cannot be tolerated by most people. The main side affect is cardiac arrest, but your tests show that you have a very strong heart. Therefore, we can use the strongest drug in your case."

"You've got to be kidding," Ariena said, not attempting to hide her shocked disbelief. "Cardiac arrest is the main *side* affect?"

"I would have thought cardiac arrest would be better described as somewhat more final than a side affect," Scott added.

"It says here that you are an athlete," Dr Price commented, looking at the file again. "An athlete's heart is normally much stronger due to the person being physically active, therefore it is unlikely that the drug would affect your heart. The other side affects can be uncomfortable but can be treated with other drugs to alleviate the symptoms. Your hair will fall out, as with any chemotherapy, but you can get a wig for free from the cancer society."

Ariena's mouth dropped open. "What?"

"I see you have lovely hair," the younger woman said, attempting to complement her, "But, don't worry it will grow back again."

*She's finally seen me,* Ariena thought. "It's not about the hair," she muttered, still shocked.

"How long will it take for this course of chemotherapy?" Scott asked.

"Again, because of it's strength, there needs to be a two week recovery period between each dose. The first course will take six months to complete, there will be a two month recovery time before the second course is started."

Ariena shook her head. "I've been told that I only have six months to live," she said.

"That's the very reason why you need the strongest possible treatment.This may give you another six months."

"And I'm supposed to spend it having chemotherapy, which will make me feel sick, my hair will fall out and I may have a heart attack?" Ariena said in disbelief.

"There is always a possibility that the treatment will give you longer, perhaps even years. We can only do everything possible. With chemotherapy and radiation, there's a chance we may slow the cancer down considerably, but there are no guarantees." She looked at her watch and said abruptly, "I can't answer any more questions. All you need to do is decide which of the two chemo-therapy treatments you will choose to have. You can read the details of both on the information I've given you and let the nurse know before you leave. The treatment will be started next week and will be done in your local hospital. Our nurse will phone you tomorrow with the date and time of your first appointment."

Ariena stood in shocked silence. Her son had stopped writing. The oncologist did not notice their reaction. "Due to the severity of the cancer that you have," she said, "and therefore the urgency for immediate treatment, we are recommending that the radiation be done during the first two week break between chemotherapy doses. Your radiologist will explain that procedure." She took a step toward the door. "I believe you have an appointment with her this afternoon?" she said. Ariena nodded. "Good," she said, opening the door. Turning to Ariena she said, "Don't worry about anything, you'll be fine. If you have any more questions, please ask the nurse. She can also help you fill out the form that you'll need to sign for the treatment." She walked out ahead of them and down the corridor.

*

Ariena and Scott looked at each other. "I can't believe that," Ariena finally said.

"Yeah, incredible," Scott concurred. The receptionist was walking towards them with a woman following close behind. She stopped at the door and pointed back up the hallway. "That way," she said to them. They stepped past her and started walking slowly together.

"Did you feel that?" Scott asked.

"You mean the number being stamped on my back?" Ariena replied.

"Yeah. Feels like we're on a factory line."

"We are," she said. "What do you reckon we should do?"

"Get off it," she replied. "We're going straight out the front door."

"I'm with you on that," he said.

They walked in silence across the parking lot, too shocked to say anything. Sitting in the car, looking out the windscreen at the building they had just walked out of, Ariena shook her head. "It's huge," she said. Scott looked at her questioningly. "The building," she said pointing in that direction, "it's huge."

"I thought you meant the whole cancer thing," he said.

"I do," she replied. "Just looking at the Clinic though, the size of the building tells you how huge the cancer industry is."

"Interesting analogy," he commented, looking at the building, "but you're right, it is an industry."

"I was reading the stats on cancer in general, and on the amount of money spent on research into the so-called cure for cancer," Ariena said, still looking at the building. "Do you know that for over 30 years they have been doing research and are no closer to finding a cure now than they were then? Since 1971, there have been multi billions of dollars supposedly spent on trying to find the cure for cancer, there's been more money raised through cancer fundraising events than for any other cause. The cancer industry is the biggest moneymaking industry in the world," she said, "and you can be sure they're not searching for a cure."

"No, that would put an end to the industry wouldn't it," he agreed.

"The way I see it," she pondered, "is that the only research that is being done, is to develop the strongest possible treatment that will keep a person sick but not kill them outright. One thing is for sure, they're not advocating eliminating the cause, not while they can continue to treat the symptoms and keep the industry alive."

"...and to keep the patients alive for as long as possible," Scott added. "Every treatment must rack up the dollars."

"The last numbers I heard put it at around $17,000 per treatment of chemo, depending on what type is used," Ariena said. "and with new drugs being developed all the time, the cost keeps going up. The calculation doesn't bear thinking about."

"...and people think it's free," he said.

"That's part of the insidiousness of the industry," she agreed, "that and the fear tactics used to make people step up onto the factory line at their lowest moment. Once they're on, they can't get off."

"Yeah." Scott nodded in agreement.

Ariena put the keys in the ignition and started the car.

"Where are we going?"

"I'm going to turn the car around so we can eat without looking at that," she said nodding towards the building, "we only have half an hour before radiologist appointment, might as well enjoy our lunch."

"Good idea." Scott reached for the bag on the back seat. "Nice wall," he observed with a smile, looking at the changed view through the windscreen.

"You can always climb over a wall," Ariena said.

"...or run through it," he added, "I've seen you do that a few times."

"Yes, the good old marathon wall," she said, remembering the times when she thought she could not go on during a marathon race, but managed to find the will to do so. "This cancer challenge is not much different," she mused, "just have to find a way through that wall."

"Yes," he agreed, munching on an apple. "This wall might be a little higher to climb and harder to run through, but you can do it. *We* can do it," he emphasised. He passed her an apple. "Better have this," he said smiling, "keep 'you know who' away."

"There's more truth in that than anything else I've heard today," Ariena replied.

*

The radiology waiting room was empty when they walked in. Within a few minutes an attractive young woman approached them and introduced herself as the radiologist.

"Hello, I'm Marita, I'd like to explain the radiation procedure to you and give you my recommendations," she said politely. "Please come into my office," she said, inviting them to follow her. Scott raised his eyebrows appreciatively. Ariena smiled at him and winked, shaking her head slightly. The radiologist's office was bright and airy, a window stood open and the sheer curtain fluttered in the breeze. The walls were painted a pale blue, the three turquoise upholstered chairs in the room toned in beautifully. On the desk stood a framed photo of a tiny puppy.

"Please make yourselves comfortable," Marita said with a smile, "I'll be with you in just a moment." As she left the room, Ariena's son said, "Cute."

"The puppy or the girl?" his mother asked. "The puppy of course," he replied. "What was the head shake for?"

"To let you know that just because she's cute doesn't mean we'll agree to anything she says," she answered.

"Hee, hee," he laughed. "Right, gotcha. She's certainly different to the last one," he added.

"Different approach for different strokes," she commented.

"Do I detect a note of cynicism?"

She raised one eyebrow at him. "We'll see," was all she said.

The radiologist explained the radiation procedure and answered all their questions in a congenial manner. "In your case, I see that you are physically fit and otherwise in good health," she commented referring to the file.

*Here we go again*, Ariena thought.

"You're even an athlete," Marita noted, looking up at Ariena. "That's great, what's your sport?"

"I run," Ariena said.

"Great," she repeated. "Short or long distance?"

"I'm an endurance athlete," Ariena replied. "Long distance, marathons and ultras."

"Wow, I'm impressed," Marita said. "I've always wanted to run a marathon. How many have you done?"

Ariena smiled. "A few," she said, glancing at her son who raised his eyebrows. "I don't consider myself a competitive runner," she clarified. "I prefer to run in nature, on mountain trails or along the beach. I like to challenge myself with the hardest and roughest terrain I can find."

"Wow," Marita said again. "That's why you're in such great shape. Physically I mean. That will serve you well through your current health problems, athletes like yourself generally recover from treatment much faster than others," she added.

"Yes," Ariena nodded. "This will be the biggest challenge so far, I'm sure. Certainly the hardest and roughest terrain."

"Exactly," Marita agreed. "Well, I like your attitude, good to consider having cancer a challenge. I think you would be a perfect candidate for a study that we are currently doing," she added with enthusiasm. Ariena looked at her but said nothing. "In the years that radiation has been used for cancer treatment, there hasn't been much change in the protocol," she explained. "The latest development has been using a laser to direct the radiation more accurately, so that the possibility of affecting other organs is lessened. Although in your case," she deferred, "with there being wide spread growth throughout the chest wall, the radiation will affect your heart and lung, but only minimally."

"That sounds encouraging," Ariena said wryly.

"At least with the laser, it will only be a small corner of the lung which wont have any adverse effect on it's functional capacity. We wont know how the heart will be affected, it will depend on how deep we need to go with the radiation," Marita explained, "but with your physical strength, that shouldn't be a concern either," she smiled. Ariena glanced towards her son. He appeared to be studying the photo of the dog. "Anyway," the radiologist said with an excited tone in her voice, "considering everything, you would be perfect for this new study."

"What is this study supposed to achieve?" Scott asked, still looking at the photo.

"It's to determine how deep we can go before affecting the other organs adversely."

"That sounds like fun," Ariena said, not attempting to take the cynicism out of her voice. "So, you want me to be a guinea pig, so to speak. Human experimentation, in other words."

"Well, I wouldn't put it quite like that," Marita replied, appearing somewhat taken aback. "The study results will help determine the best dosage for many other people in the future," she ventured.

"Sacrifice my health to save others," Ariena clarified.

"Well, I wouldn't say *sacrifice*," she replied.

"What would you say?" Ariena challenged her. "Isn't that what is happening to millions of guinea pigs, and other animals, in the name of research? After all, with what happens to them during their so-called lives as experimental animals, they're destined to die anyway. Is that the reason you think I'm a perfect candidate for this study? Because I'm going to die of cancer anyway?"

The young woman looked devastated. "I'm sorry," she said, "no of course not. It's because you are strong and otherwise healthy. You'll have more chance of withstanding the affects of the radiation than most."

"I've heard this reasoning before," Ariena said. "I fail to see that deliberately compromising vital organs can be beneficial to anyone. I'm sorry, but I wont be participating in any study or treatment that will compromise my body any further than it already is."

"OK, you don't have to be on the study if you're not willing to take that risk," the radiologist said, "the radiation treatment that is scheduled for you otherwise will be much less aggressive."

"Marita," Ariena said, looking directly at her, "I believe you are in this job because you are genuinely concerned about other people's health, that is commendable. However, have you ever considered the consequences of what you are doing, not only to others, but also to yourself. Being exposed to radiation as a radiologist is a high risk factor in itself."

"Yes, thank you for your concern," she replied politely, "obviously I am aware of the risks regarding radiology. However, we're here to discuss your treatment for cancer, and radiation has been considered an effective treatment for many years."

"Radiation has been *used* as a treatment for cancer for many years," Ariena countered, "from my research there is little evidence that it is effective in any way, other than adversely. There has been no improvement in the technology since it was first experimented with, apart from being able to direct the radiation more accurately with the laser. In my opinion, it is still an experiment, a compromising, debilitating and barbaric practice, legalised for human experimentation." Scott stared at his mother.

"I'm, I'm sorry you feel that way," Marita stammered, looking a little shaken. "Um, does that mean…" her question trailed off and hung in the air.

"That I wont be having radiation?" Ariena finished it for her. "Yes, that's exactly what it means."

"I'm sorry to hear that," she said looking somewhat crestfallen.

"I'm not," Scott said.

Ariena smiled at him. "I'm sorry to see an obviously compassionate girl like you in this compromising situation," she said to the radiologist. "This conversation has been most enlightening, I hope perhaps it has been for you too. It has certainly given me the information I needed to make an informed choice about my life. You might want to consider your own life and change your job to something more positive," she suggested with a smile.

"I do admire your courage," the young woman smiled back at her, "and thank you for your concern. However, I've spent over eight years studying and working in this capacity. It's too late to change my career now. Don't worry, I'll be careful," she added.

"It's never too late to change for the better," Ariena replied, "just watch me."

\*

"How's the research going, Mum?" Scott asked as he let himself in.

"It's going," she replied looking up at him and smiling. "We've checked into all the details on the chemo that was recommended, makes for very scary reading!"

"No doubt," he said, "it's scary stuff. Heard from the Clinic today?"

"Oh, yes," she replied. "They haven't missed calling every day since we were there. I've told them that I haven't decided yet and that I'll get back to them, but they insist on trying to get me to agree to the treatment over the phone. I've explained that I'm doing more research until I'm absolutely satisfied with my decision, and that it will take time. I've asked them not to call me, that I'll call them when I've made my decision, but they keep calling and telling me I don't have time, that if I delay any more it will be too late."

"That's using fear tactics," Scott said. "You don't need that. Sounds like harassment calls to me, tell them you'll lodge a complaint, maybe they'll stop calling."

"I'm trying not to let it get to me," Ariena replied, "but it is quite upsetting. Yesterday, it was the oncologist who phoned, I guess the nurse must have told her that I was difficult to persuade. Anyway, it was good because I could ask her a few questions about some of the research I'd been doing. When I mentioned a couple of studies that I'd found in the medical journal and asked if she was aware of the stats from those studies, do you know what she said?"

"Go on, tell me."

"She said that she doesn't have time to read the medical journal, she's too busy with her patients."

"…and what did you say?"

"I said, 'doesn't that tell you something? Isn't there something wrong with the picture, if the oncologists don't have time to update themselves on developments in their field because they are too busy with so many patients?' I said that clearly what they were doing wasn't working and that would be all the more reason for them to be looking into other solutions."

"What was her response to that?"

"She just said, 'we're too overwhelmed.' I told her that is because she's working in a self perpetuating industry, not a health related system. Do you know, she was not aware that the company that formulates chemotherapy treatments produces the chemicals used to make carcinogenic pesticides also."

"What was her reaction to that?"

"She said that the production of the treatments was not her concern. She said she is an oncologist, she deals with people, not production. She honestly didn't get the connection!"

"Yeah, it's amazing. They don't want to know, it would put their careers at stake. I'm sure they originally got into it from a personal perspective of wanting to help people, but the sickness industry is not run by the carers, it's run by money-motivated corporations who are in the business of keeping people sick, and cancer is the biggest moneymaker of all. This is big business, the pharmaceutical industry is in control here, not the caregivers."

"Yes, it's sad, tragic really," she commented, "but I'll not be dragged into it uninformed. Their fear tactics wont sway me from making my own informed decisions."

"So, where are you at with her now?"

"I asked her yesterday if I could get a second opinion on the recommendations."

"I bet that went down well," Scott said, smiling at his mother.

"Actually, she was OK with it. She reminded me that the recommendations came as a result of the group of oncologists at the Clinic, but she said there were at least nine other cancer specialists in the country whom I could see. Of course, she also reminded me that I should consider that it would take more time to get appointments, and that time is of the essence in my case."

"So, what's the plan?"

"I asked her to set up a conference call with all nine specialists and herself," she replied.

"Are you serious?" Scott looked aghast at his mother.

"She asked me that too," Ariena replied, "and my answer was yes. The nurse phoned today to confirm the call is set for tomorrow morning, 9 o'clock."

"Excellent," he said, "you do know that they'll all say the same thing though," he warned.

"Maybe, but at least I'll have a chance to ask a few more questions that they may be able to answer," she said. "I'm sure I'll have a few more since I have an appointment to see the naturopathic physician this afternoon."

"Oh, good," he responded with a smile. "Take all the notes with you that we made about their recommendations. I'm sure he'll be interested in all your research too."

\*

Ariena sat by the roaring fire, drinking a cup of herbal tea. The naturopath's waiting room was warm and welcoming, with the smell and ambiance of the wood fire, the aroma of herbal tea, and the floral upholstered chairs comfortably arranged around the room. A rack of magazines with topics on gardening, animal and bird watching, baby and child care and natural remedies, hung on the wall beside a large painting of wild lavender. A basket of fresh apples sat on a low, hand hewn wooden table in the centre of the room.

Ariena watched as an elderly couple entered the room from outside.

"It's getting cold out there," the old man said, "lovely to be in here though," he grinned. Ariena looked around at everyone in the room, they were all smiling. *What a contrast*, she thought to herself, recalling the cold, sterile waiting rooms that she'd recently experienced, with anxious, worried people sitting awkwardly on hard plastic chairs.

\*

"Good morning everyone," the young doctor said brightly as he entered the room, "nice and cosy in here." He bent down and looked at the fire. "That log will keep burning for a while," he said and turning to the elderly couple he patted the old man on the knee. "Now if it's not warm enough for you, don't hesitate to throw another log on the fire and help yourselves to an apple everyone, they're the last off the old tree out back, don't look much, but they're really delicious." The old man stood up and went over to the table. He picked up the basket of apples and walked around the room, offering them to each person.

"I think it's a ploy to keep us all away," he said jokingly, "the good doctor knows what's best for us."

Dressed in an open neck plaid shirt and linen trousers, his beard clipped short and hair falling to his broad shoulders, Dr Wright stepped lightly into the room. In his hand he held two glasses and a jug of water, lemon slices floating gaily on top. He placed the glasses on the table and filled them with water. Passing a glass to Ariena, he sat down on the chair opposite her. The only thing missing from the doctor's consulting room was a fireplace. The padded chairs were set around a small table in one corner, a large wooden desk was pushed up against the wall on the other side of the room. A bright yellow vase held an arrangement of autumn leaves on the table. Dainty lace curtains hung in the window, framing a tranquil scene, the old apple tree, bare of it's leaves, standing naked in a leafy carpet of gold.

\*

"You look great," he said smiling at her.

She smiled back. "It's a disguise," she said, taking a sip of water. "Did they send over my file?"

"I received a report from your family doctor," he replied, "but I believe there's been other developments since then?"

"Yes, I had surgery," Ariena answered, "against my better judgement I believe," she added. "They removed the tumour and lymph nodes, also against my wishes I might add." She looked at him with a wry smile. "It's been confirmed," she said, "I have what they call a highly aggressive cancer that is apparently spreading rapidly. The prognosis is that I may have about six months before the cancer is spread throughout my body. The oncologist is recommending chemotherapy and radiation. They want to get started on the treatment immediately. They're phoning me constantly, telling me I don't have time to think about it or do any research of my own. It's like they're using scare tactics to get me to make decisions out of fear."

Ariena put her glass down on the table and wrung her hands together. Dr Wright reached across the table and took her hands in his.

"They say the chemo may give me another six months," she looked at him, tears welling in her eyes. He stood up, walked around the table, reaching his arms out to her. She rose and stepped into his arms, a sob escaping from her throat. He held her for a few moments, then stepped back, his hands still steadying her shoulders.

"Have you decided what you're going to do?" he asked, his voice gruff with emotion.

"Not yet," she said, wiping the tears from her cheeks, "that's why I'm here. I want your opinion on everything, and your advice on what I should do." She smiled at him, and sat down as he returned to his chair.

"Ariena, I can't give my opinion or my advice until I've fully studied all the reports," he said, "but what I can tell you now is this. No matter what you decide, no matter what the outcome, and, no matter how hard the journey," he looked into her tearful eyes, "I will walk all the way with you. I will give you whatever advice and information I can to help you make your own decisions, and I will support whatever your decisions with the best of my knowledge and ability," he took her hands again and held them.

"Thank you," she said, "I know you will. Like I said, that's why I'm here."

He squeezed her hands and reached for a pen and notepaper. "Well, let's make a plan," he said, "what were your first thoughts about the diagnosis?"

"I guess I couldn't believe it," Ariena replied, "the surgeon said I was in denial, but it was more like I was shocked and astounded that it could happen to me. I mean, I've always been healthy and active, I've never eaten junk food and I've been vegetarian most of my life. I've never taken drugs, not even an aspirin! I don't smoke or even drink alcohol," she looked a him with a smile, "apart from the odd glass of wine, but it has to be the best French wine though." She laughed at the irony of it.

"What were your thoughts once you did believe it," he asked, "once it had really sunk in?"

"I was angry," she said without hesitation, "I was angry and sad and scared all at once."

"...and now? What are your thoughts now?" he asked smiling at her candidness.

"Now? Now I feel like it's a challenge," she said, "like I can beat it. I know I can," she said nodding. "I just have to get rid of those moments of doubt and fear so I can get on with it." She looked at him, smiling as he was writing notes on the paper. "You're right," she said, "I need a plan, a plan of action, not distraction. I need to take control of my own health and not feel as if I'm being pushed into making decisions that I might regret, or doing things that I don't believe in."

The doctor sat back. "There you are," he said with a laugh, "I knew you wouldn't be too far away."

She sat back too and smiled broadly at him. "What were the notes you were writing?" she asked.

"Ah, that's my grocery list," he said with a smirk.

"Oh, you're good," she said, "you're very good." They both laughed.

"I have been doing a great deal of thinking about the 'why me' side of things," Ariena continued, "because I was sure that there had to be an overriding factor that caused the cancer. When I was really little, I did have some of the usual 'childhood sickness' like measles, mumps and chickenpox, but I always got over them really quickly. According to my mother, I also had scarlet fever, but since the age of three, I've never been chronically sick, I've never even had a cold! So, I figured it wouldn't have been a nutritional deficiency. Therefore, I tried to think of anytime in my life that my body might have been compromised, by either physical or emotional trauma, and I did come up with a couple of reasons that may have been contributing factors. I recall two incidents at school that involved physical trauma, one was when I was punched in the chest, about the time when my breasts were just starting to develop, the other was when I was knocked out cold during athletics when another kid and I literally ran into each other head-on! I was so winded that it felt like my lungs had collapsed! I remember having chest pains for a couple of weeks after that."

"Sounds like you were playing rough! How did you get punched?"

"I really can't remember how it happened to be honest," she said, "but I do remember the pain in my breast lasted for a while then too."

"You mentioned emotional trauma," he prompted.

"Yes," she replied, " I realise that breast cancer could well be triggered by a hormonal imbalance or traumatic emotional stress which could create the imbalance. Since I've never had any problems with an imbalance and menstruation has always been normal etc, I tried to think of any emotional incident or stress that I'd had. Apart from what I would consider normal for everyone, especially women, wives and mothers," she said with a smile, "I have not ever considered myself to be 'stressed out' so to speak. There has never been any major emotional trauma such as sudden death in the family or anything like that. However, there were a few times, as a woman, a wife and a mother, when emotions gave way to tears and I've cried uncontrollably."

"Have there been times when you've been so upset that you wanted to cry, but didn't? Times when you've held back the tears?" he asked.

"Oh, yes," she said nodding, "too many, I'm sure."

"Not crying when you need to certainly causes more emotional stress than crying, which does help to release the immediate stress," he said.

"I never really thought I was depressed or anything like that, I just thought that it happened to everyone, again, especially as a wife and mother," she added.

"It most likely does," he agreed, "but that doesn't mean it's not emotionally damaging to your health."

"Exactly," she agreed, "and it all builds up over time, so I'm assuming what most women like myself think is normal, is possibly doing damage that may manifest as cancer later in life."

"Yes," he said, "emotional stress can have a cumulative affect on one's health if it is not addressed."

"Well, anyway," she continued, "while I was thinking of all these incidences, I noticed that I felt a bit sad at times, so I realised that there's more to it than just the incidences themselves. I realised that the mere act of thinking can cause emotional stress depending on what your thoughts are about."

"Absolutely," he agreed, "that's where the toxic effect comes in. Emotions such as sorrow, sadness, grief, guilt, jealousy, anger, hate and fear, all have a highly toxic effect on the body, and like I said, if these are not addressed, the toxic effect builds up over time, creating symptoms of dis-ease in the body, like anxiety and depression."

"When you say 'addressed' you mean 'dealing with' the situation?" she asked.

"Yes," he replied, "for instance, sorrow, sadness and grief, depending on what has caused the emotion, may be eased by doing calming therapy or having counselling; whereas guilt, jealousy, anger and hate require reasoning, forgiveness and love."

"Fear of course is the big one," Ariena said, "eliminating fear requires all the above and more."

"Indeed," he agreed.

"Anyway," she continued, " I got to thinking that if emotional stress can cause a toxic effect in the body, then what about all the environmental toxins that we're exposed to everyday, in the home, at work, or just walking down the street."

"Those are toxic substances that can enter the body when we breathe, eat and drink, and through our skin," he said, "so they don't create a toxic effect, they *are* a toxic affect. Most of these substances are completely foreign to the body and are very difficult to eliminate from the system. So again, over time they accumulate in the body and eventually go into overload. That is when a person becomes symptomatic, because the body is not at ease. Symptoms are messages from the body telling us that it is in a state of dis-ease, and they can range from a mild headache to a cancerous tumour."

"Yes, so I thought about any time in my life that I may have been exposed to any highly toxic substances and remembered immediately about two major incidents," Ariena said. "About eight years ago I was painting our boat with anti-fouling, you know the paint that is used to kill barnacles or stop them from attaching to the bottom of the boat, it's extremely toxic for that reason. Well, I had a can of it open in my hand when I fell from the scaffolding and poured the whole can over myself as I went down!"

Dr Wright raised his eyebrows in shock and stared at her. "You're kidding," he exclaimed.

"Nope, unfortunately not," she replied, "that paint went all over me. It completely covered my skin, went through my hair and into my ears, up my nose and into my mouth, and I know I swallowed some!"

"It's a wonder that didn't kill you outright," he said.

"I know," she agreed, "just shows you how resilient the body is. I remember telling the doctor at the hospital not to use turps to remove it because I thought it would burn my skin. I wasn't thinking about the toxic effect the paint was already having as it soaked through the skin and into my system. I think they used kerosene to remove most of it, but it took two to three months for my skin to return to its normal colour, not to mention my hair! The worst was that I could taste and smell it for weeks!"

"Well, that would most definitely have a major toxic effect on your body," the doctor said, still appearing shocked. "Did you sustain any injuries from the fall?"

"My elbow was dislocated which tore all the ligaments and tendons," Ariena replied, and chuckled as she said, "it wasn't the fall that hurt, it was the stopping at the end!" The doctor burst out laughing. Putting his hand over his mouth, he apologised in muffled tones, "I'm sorry, that wasn't very professional," continuing to chuckle.

"It was even funnier if you'd seen what I looked like when I walked into the hospital," she said, laughing at herself, "just picture it; I was limping on both feet, ever seen that? it's a good trick, my arm was hanging at a weird angle, I was covered from head to toe in dripping paint, but get this, the paint was white and so was my bikini!" He broke into laughter again, shaking his head as he tried to stop.

"I was moaning because everything hurt and I must have looked and sounded like a ghost or apparition as I came through the automatic opening doors, because the nurses threw their hands up in horror when they saw me!" she said, laughing herself. He reached for the water and filled their glasses, still trying to control his laughter. She reached for her glass, raised it saying, "Cheers, here's to seeing the funny side of it!"

"I don't suppose the actual incident was, but that was hilarious the way you told it," he said.

"Nope, it sure wasn't funny at the time," she replied, still smiling. He took a few more sips of water to regain his composure.

"You said there were two major incidents where you were exposed to highly toxic substances," he reminded her, "what was the other one? I hope you didn't do that again?"

"No," Ariena assured him, "the other was a case of being in the wrong place at the wrong time. It certainly was not within my control to prevent or avoid it." She looked at him soberly.

"Go on," he said, looking at her seriously.

"One word," she said, "Chernobyl."

"You were there?" he asked in an astonished tone.

"Not at ground zero," she replied, "but right in the path of the fallout. We were living in France at the time, the fallout came right over the country before it headed north."

"You could see it?" he was still astounded.

"You could see it and you could smell it," she replied, "that's what alerted us that there was something wrong. We knew nothing of the disaster at that point. We just noticed that the sky turned a grayish green and the air became very heavy, a bit like when there is a big storm brewing around dusk, but it was morning so it became very eerie as it darkened the sky." Her face became serious as she recalled that fateful day. "We had seen something like it once before, when a storm was rolling in late in the day, so we went outside to look. Then we smelt it." She looked at him and slowly shook her head. "Something told me this was not the weather, I felt a warning feeling inside and my heart started pounding. I didn't know what it was, but fear had enveloped me, so I instinctively rushed the children inside and shut the doors and windows. It took about an hour before the sky started to clear and the day became bright again, and by that time we'd heard on the radio about the nuclear disaster."

"Wow, there must have been hundreds, maybe thousands of people affected by the fallout," he commented. "What happened after that day?"

"We had no obvious signs or symptoms, although I remember having a metallic taste in my mouth for a while. The French authorities set up a program of washing the field crops as they were harvested, they used high pressure hoses with water and I think they added some kind of detergent or bleach to the wash," Ariena recalled, "but we stopped eating any fresh produce and bought veggies and fruit in a can that had a production date before the day of the disaster. Ironic isn't it," she pondered, "to think it would be safer to eat out of a can, but we did. The washing program only last a couple of weeks, which doesn't make any sense since there were still crops in the ground, especially when you consider that the people doing the washing were clothed in anti toxic suits and masks so they looked like astronauts. When you think about it, not only were the existing crops contaminated but the ground too, so future crops would have been affected as well."

"For years, I would think," he agreed, "if you consider that to have a certified organic farm the soil needs to have no toxic substances on or in it for at least seven years, imagine how long it must take for the soil to regenerate after having had nuclear fallout."

"Yes, I'm sure we'll only just start to hear about incidents with people's health now and in the future," she said, "and how many people will realise it may have been due to exposure?"

"Of course, there will be thousands of people who are not noticeably affected," he added, "so the correlation may never be fully realised."

"Exactly," she agreed, "I'm sure it would depend on how high a person's toxic load was at the time too. Perhaps if I had not already been compromised by the paint incident and other emotional toxic build up, then it may not have reached a maximum and gone into overload for me either."

"You're right," he agreed, "but eventually something would tip the scales and it would manifest into ill health or dis-ease in your body, but most people would not look back to establish what may have caused a health issue. Once they become symptomatic, they just want to eliminate the discomfort of the symptoms, and that's where the medical protocol of treating the symptoms comes in," he added. "Unfortunately, it never addresses the underlying cause, so their symptoms become chronic and they are permanently in a state of varying degrees of ill health."

*

"Yes, and it appears to me that most of the treatments are worse than the symptoms, or at least they create a worsening state of health, which then requires more treatment," she said, "it's ongoing and it just doesn't make sense. So that's why I wanted to establish what the most likely cause or causes could be for me to have a diagnosis of cancer, so I can eliminate the cause," she reasoned, "because if I don't do that, and just treat the symptoms, the cancer will eventually recur or manifest elsewhere or in another form."

"It's good that you've taken the time to think about this," Dr

Wright said, "so what do you propose to do about it, now that you believe you have established the cause?"

"Well, if I have a high toxic load, which it would appear I must have considering my health history," Ariena replied, "then clearly I need to lower it somehow. Once it's low enough for the body to start rejuvenating and healing, I need to continue thinking consciously about my lifestyle and be constantly aware of making the right choices, so I can maintain a state of optimal health."

"Excellent," he said approvingly, "you are absolutely right in your reasoning. Do you have any idea what you could do to achieve that?"

"I've heard that the far infrared rays from the sun will eliminate heavy toxins," Ariena said, "so I've been researching that and considering the urgency, it would appear that using an infrared sauna would be the best bet, since it's safe to use twice a day, getting enough safe sunshine may not be as easy. I'll definitely start doing that, and try to get in the sun early in the morning whenever I can as well. Do you have any other suggestions?"

"Yes," he said, "there is a treatment called chelation, which has an intravenous protocol and is specifically for lowering the toxic load. We can do that here along with immune therapy. You should have a live blood analyses done to determine your toxic load before you start. It's incredibly accurate and will give you a good picture, literally, of the type of toxic buildup you have, as well as where and when it started accumulating. There are also several blood, urine and saliva tests that will help determine how we establish your immune therapy protocol, we can start doing those when you come in for your first immune therapy."

Dr Wright paused a moment before adding, "It would also be very helpful for you to have a PET scan done if you decide to go ahead with chemo treatment."

"A PET scan? Doesn't that use nuclear medicine imaging?"

"Yes, but PET scans can show up a cancer, it can reveal the stage of the cancer and show whether the cancer has spread as well as indicating the effectiveness of ongoing chemotherapy."

"You know I'm not happy about having agreed to the surgery that I've had already, and I'm not keen on the idea of having chemo," Ariena confided in him, "I've already refused the radiation because it just doesn't make sense to compromise the body further by poisoning and burning it. So to me, a PET scan is radiation personified!"

"Certainly doesn't fit into the 'do no harm' creed that we go by," the young doctor agreed.

"I understand the theory behind using chemo because it literally kills everything in it's path, so the idea that it will kill the cancer cells is one thing, but it's also going to kill all the good cells too," Ariena reasoned. "How is the body supposed to recover from that when it's already compromised?"

"That's why the chemo treatment is given in stages with recovery time in between," he explained. "A full dose would kill you outright, and has done in some cases by causing cardiac arrest," he added.

"I know," she said, "the oncologist called that a side effect! My concern with that, apart from the obvious, is that as an athlete, my rested heart rate is already very low. Having a sudden severe toxic overload from the chemo causing cardiac arrest when the heart rate is so low would be fatal for sure," she said, shaking her head.

"There may be a way around that," the doctor said, "if the chemo dose is lowered and the effectiveness is more precise." He reached for a file on his desk. Opening it he continued, "There is a complementary therapy that is used alongside chemotherapy to make it more effective, it's called IPT-Insulin Potentiation Therapy. I have information on IPT here from one of the clinics where it is widely used, would you like me to read it?"

"Yes, please," Ariena replied, "it sounds very interesting." The doctor took a page out of the file and started to read.

"IPT, also known as low dose chemotherapy, is one of the safest and most innovative approaches to treating cancer. It is a kinder, gentler way to fight cancer effectively, including particularly aggressive cancers, but is also effective on a wide variety of cancer types. IPT is also believed to help detoxify. While IPT kills cancer cells, it flushes toxins into the circulation, enabling them to leave the body. The use of insulin also assists debilitated cancer patients with appetite and metabolism, helping to mitigate the wasting that accompanies the disease and its treatment. This alternative treatment has almost none of the side effects such as nausea, radical hair loss, liver damage, and DNA distortion that is seen routinely with standard chemotherapy."

"Sold right there," Ariena commented.

"Thought you'd say that," he said smiling at her. "This explains how it works," he continued.

"The key to IPT as a cancer cure is the body's own hormone, insulin. Insulin manages the delivery of glucose across cell membranes into the cells. Cancer cells have 10-20 times more insulin receptors on their surface than normal cells. When insulin is released into the bloodstream by the pancreas in response to a meal, the insulin attaches to these receptors on the surface of the cell and opens channels in the cell wall to allow nutrients to go into the cell. Because cancer cells have more of these receptors, they compete for food more successfully than normal cells. In this way, cancer cells thrive and normal cells are compromised."

\*

"I never knew that, about the receptors," Ariena exclaimed, "makes total sense."

"Yes," he agreed, "you may have heard the expression that sugar feeds cancer? Well, indeed it does, and that extreme need for sugar is used to advantage with IPT when treating cancer. For example, PET scans find cancer by looking at the sugar uptake. The radioactive agent is mixed with sugar water and, because cancer cells take up much more sugar than normal cells, the radioactive agent congregates in the cancer cells. The resulting picture will indicate enhanced uptake and a mass where the cancer is," he explained, "but with IPT, instead of using a radioactive agent along with the sugar, chemotherapy is used, and the cellular membranes are opened for significantly better absorption."

"That makes sense too," she said, "and better than using radioactive agents, they make you glow in the dark!"

"Hence the reason it's called nuclear medicine," he said, then resumed reading from his notes.

"In IPT, insulin is administered to trigger a drop in the patient's blood sugar level. Healthy cells shift over to fat metabolism, but cancer cells rely almost entirely on sugar metabolism, so they go into an emergency mode and open all of their membranes to get the sugar they need. At this point, a small amount of chemotherapy is administered (about one-tenth the amount of standard chemotherapy dose is used), followed quickly by glucose (sugar). The cancer cells, in their effort to get the glucose, take in almost the entire dose of chemotherapy drugs as well. The drugs poison and eventually kill the cancer cells."

"Wow, that's a huge difference in the dosage," Ariena commented.

"Yes," the doctor replied, "and this method targets the cytotoxic drugs directly to the cancer cell. There is little chemo left over to cause a toxic reaction within healthy cells so patients who treat cancer with IPT have far fewer side effects. Whereas with standard chemotherapy, insulin is not used to open the cells. That's why patients must be given a large dose of drugs so that enough will be absorbed by the cells to do the job. The majority of the drugs are not taken up by the cancer cells so the massive dosage wreaks havoc to healthy cells and blood components. Because standard chemotherapy does not target cancer cells, the immune system takes a beating and patients experience many unpleasant side effects."

"That's putting it mildly," she said.

He smiled and continued reading.

"In IPT, the word potentiate means that one substance; insulin, enhances the effectiveness of another substance; chemotherapy, and therefore less drugs are needed. Simply put, IPT consists of a pulse of hypoglycemia (low blood sugar) that improves the effectiveness of therapeutic drugs and supports health. IPT makes cell membranes more permeable, increasing the uptake of drugs into cells and helps transport drugs across the blood-brain barrier. Along with its ability to help deliver higher levels of the chemo-therapy drugs into the cancer cells, insulin also causes these cells to go into their growth phase where they become more vulnerable to the chemotherapy drugs. The cells are hit harder at a time when they are most vulnerable to the assault, thus maximising results. A study conducted at George Washington University showed that the chemo drug, methotrexate, when used with insulin, increased the drug's cell-killing effect by a factor of 10,000."

"That's incredible," Ariena exclaimed.

"Isn't it," he agreed, "and that's obviously why the dosage has to be lowered to one-tenth."

"Absolutely crucial I would think," she said.

"Yes, and that could be a problem," he said, "getting the oncologist to agree to lowering the dose."

"But lowering the dose would make it safer, with or without

the insulin," she commented, "so what could they have against trying it?"

"The answer to that question is right here," he said, turning to read the last paragraph.

"IPT's innovative approach was developed in the 1920s, but was first used for cancer in 1945. The practice of IPT is now worldwide, but it is not yet taught in America's conventional medical schools however, and of course, pharmaceutical companies do not look favourably upon IPT because it uses so little of their product."

"Right, back to the pharmaceutical companies and their multi billion dollar sickness industry," Ariena said, shaking her head in disbelief. "They're not concerned with the patient's quality of life, no matter how short or long it may be. We're just numbers and percentages, we're just statistics," she said.

"Yes, well, there you have it," he said, "but the natural approach differs from the conventional approach. We recognise that each person is unique, and each person will respond differently to different therapies. That is why IPT for an breast cancer patient will follow a different protocol than for a lung cancer patient or an ovarian cancer patient."

"So, IPT is the primary treatment to stop the immediate danger by halting the growth of cancer quickly," Ariena said.

"Yes, that is correct," Dr Wright confirmed, "the treatment need not be worse than the disease. If everyone were aware of IPT, no one would choose standard chemotherapy and radiation. IPT patients have much more energy and higher expectations for their recovery, and are able to devote more attention to their wellness and improving their quality of life. However, IPT sessions should also be interspersed with other natural therapies that attack the cancer cells, help the liver detoxify, and strengthen the immune system. Healing is a process, one that Mother Nature tends to go about slowly, and in layers. The goal is to eliminate the cancer you have, and then keep it from returning."

"So, what will the natural therapy protocol involve?" Ariena asked.

"We will get started on that right away," he replied, "I'll figure out a combination of intravenous treatments along with a nutritional regime that will help build the immune system. I'll also get in touch with a colleague who has experience with ITP," the doctor continued, "and get his opinion on whether you should pursue it further. Meanwhile, tell me about your research on the chemo treatment that has been recommended for you."

*

"OK," Ariena referred to her notes again, "the descriptions and side effects of the particular drugs recommended are very scary, there are four pages of contraindications, all in super small type! I've condensed that info and a few studies done on the recommended combination of treatments into this report. Shall I read it out?"

"Yes, please do," the doctor replied, "that way we can discuss points as you come to them."

"Good thing I was the last patient for the day," Ariena said, "this may take a while."

"I figured that," he said with a smile, "but it's important that we go over everything thoroughly now, so we know where we're starting from." He poured some more water into their glasses and settled back in his chair. "Go ahead when you're ready," he said.

"OK, as you know, the recommendations for my treatment are surgery, chemotherapy and radiation," Ariena said, "and because the cancer is considered highly aggressive and has already spread to the lymph nodes and chest wall, it is also recommended that I have the strongest and highest doses of chemo and radiation."

"In theory, that makes sense," he commented, "but in reality, perhaps not."

"No, in reality it makes no sense at all," agreed Ariena, "and that is because it's the same theory for everyone. A person's lifestyle is not taken into account at all, and as we know, as an athlete, both chemo and radiation could potentially be highly dangerous due to the low rested heart rate. Neither the oncologist nor the radiologist had any concept of what that meant when I mentioned it. The other very important factor that is not considered with these recommendations, is a person's nutritional needs. Apart from being told specific foods that I *cannot* eat as they would impair the results of the treatment, I have been advised what I can continue on as normal."

"Normal being the Standard American Diet we are to assume," he added.

"Yes, exactly," she agreed. "So apparently, there are certain foods that render some of the drugs that are recommended for the side effects of the chemo, completely useless. For instance if I eat grapefruit, it will counteract one of the drugs effectiveness in suppressing nausea brought on by the chemo. I've also been told not to eat or drink anything that will help build the immune system as that would be counteractive towards the chemo which will effectively shut the immune system down. Now, that was about the time that I was completely convinced that having chemo did not make any sense," she added.

"Well, the idea of the chemo is to kill as many of the cancer cells that it can," he explained, "and if you are building up the immune system, of course that will be counterproductive."

"I get that," she said, "but here's when the 'what if' comes in.

What if the chemo kills every cell in it's path and the immune system can't recover?"

"It's a gamble you take if you agree to have chemo," he replied, "and having the strongest and highest dose is even more of a gamble."

"I guess for most people, it's an easy gamble to take if you've just had the death sentence delivered to you," Ariena said.

"That is most probably the theory," he agreed, "you know, what have you got to lose?"

"Since you're already going to lose your life anyway," she said, picking up on his train of thought. "So, you become an experiment."

"It's all an experiment," he agreed, "there is no conclusive evidence that any progress is being made with this line of treatment because it does not allow the body's own system to do what it is supposed to do, and that's heal itself."

"Exactly," she said. "However, we have done extensive research into all the recommended treatments separately as well as combined, including radiotherapy even though I've already turned it down. We're keeping an open mind in case we can come up with a complimentary therapy that will assist the body to endure the treatment, recover and heal itself at the same time."

"Or do all that *and* assist the chemo in finding the cancer cells and not affecting the good cells," he added. "If the chemo can be directed to only kill the cancer cells and be eliminated from the body effectively without causing side effects, then it may have some potential benefit."

\*

"We logged on to the databases, putting in the drug names; FAC – fluorouracil ("5–FU" or 5–fluorouracil), Adriamycin, and cyclophosphamide, and CAF – cyclophosphamide, Adriamycin, and fluorouracil ("5 FU" or 5 fluorouracil), and the combinations of FAC and CAF that were recommended and it came up with almost 100,000 research papers! So we limited the search to humans, breast, and review articles, which brought it down to about a couple of thousand articles! From these we have selected a few that seem most specifically relevant, that is, larger scale trials of the FAC/CAF combination and overviews of chemo in breast cancer. One single article is really long and technical but it concludes that in this study (over 1500 women) the best option was surgery plus radiation plus the combination of chemo recommended for me, but it looks at CMF – cyclophosphamide, methotrexate, and fluorouracil ("5–FU" or 5–fluorouracil) treatment, not FAC/CAF."

"Let's have a look at it anyway," he said, "keeping in mind of course that most of these studies are funded by the pharmaceutical companies so are generally biased."

"Yes, I'm aware of that," she replied, "but some of the results and mortality rates are interesting, especially those regarding high doses. Anyway, I've taken out all the references and other data not relevant to the overall study, but have kept all that information intact in the printed version for you."

"Good, you've certainly been doing your homework," he said with a smile.

"Yes, me, *and* my family, *and* some friends. One thing is for sure, I'm not going to make any more decisions without being fully informed," she declared. "Well, here it is, I'll read it out and interject where we need to discuss anything.

"This study covers postoperative radiotherapy in high-risk premenopausal women with breast cancer who receive adjuvant chemotherapy. The abstract background states that irradiation after mastectomy can reduce locoregional recurrences in women with breast cancer, but whether it prolongs survival remains controversial.

"So, even though it's recommended, I wont be having a mastectomy. Most of the patients on this study did," Ariena said, "but the survival rate is not great with or without, which proves the instinctive theory that it doesn't make sense anyway. Having the breast removed is about as traumatic as it gets for a woman and I don't need any more trauma, emotional or otherwise."

"No," he agreed, "having the breast removed would certainly play havoc with your hormones as well, and that's something else we want to avoid. You need to bring everything into balance, not tip the scales any further."

"Anyway, to continue," she said, "a randomised trial was conducted of radiotherapy after mastectomy in high-risk premenopausal women, all of whom also received adjuvant systemic chemotherapy.

"A total of 1708 women who had undergone mastectomy for pathological stage II or III breast cancer were randomly assigned to receive eight cycles of CMF plus irradiation of the chest wall and regional lymph nodes (852 women) or nine cycles of CMF alone (856 women). The median length of follow-up was 114 months. The end points were locoregional recurrence, distant metastases, disease-free survival, and overall survival.

"The frequency of locoregional recurrence alone or with distant metastases was 9 percent among the women who received radiotherapy plus CMF and 32% among those who received CMF alone. The probability of survival free of disease after 10 years was 48% among the women assigned to radiotherapy plus CMF and 34% among those treated only with CMF. Overall survival at 10 years was 54% among those given radiotherapy and CMF and 45% among those who received CMF alone. Multivariate analysis demonstrated that irradiation after mastectomy significantly improved disease-free survival and overall survival, irrespective of tumor size, the number of positive nodes, or the histopathological grade.

"So what they're saying here, as I understand it," Ariena said, "is that those who had radiotherapy had less recurrence and metastases than those who did not, but the percentages are not high, so the majority had recurrence with or without radiation. Not only that, but the survival rate percentage was also low in both cases, being either below or only just over 50 per cent. That means close to the majority actually died."

"Yes," he agreed again, "interesting how if you put the percentages into that perspective, it tells you something quite different doesn't it?"

"Exactly," she nodded.

"Now, from this study, it was concluded that the addition of postoperative irradiation to mastectomy and adjuvant chemotherapy reduces locoregional recurrences and prolongs survival in high-risk premenopausal women with breast cancer. Randomised clinical trials have established that adjuvant chemotherapy or hormonal treatment prolongs the survival of patients with breast cancer. As a result of these studies, large numbers of women with breast cancer now receive one or both of these treatments postoperatively. A number of randomised trials have also shown that overall survival in patients with small tumors was the same whether they were treated with limited surgery plus irradiation or total mastectomy.

"So again, the argument for having a total mastectomy doesn't stand well from this study," Ariena commented, continuing to read.

"For this reason, many patients are now treated locally with conservative measures, such as lumpectomy plus axillary dissection and irradiation to residual breast tissue; some also receive adjuvant systemic therapy. Total mastectomy, however, is still the treatment of choice for many patients, especially those with more diffuse local disease. The role of radiotherapy after mastectomy has been evaluated in several randomised trials. Overall, these studies have shown a significant reduction in locoregional recurrences with postoperative irradiation but no improvement in long term survival, irrespective of nodal status.

"Hence the recommended lumpectomy and removal of lymph nodes for me," Ariena commented, "with the surgeon wanting the option of doing a mastectomy. I really don't think that it is the patients who initially choose to have a mastectomy, they get talked into it."

"Most patients wouldn't question the doctor's or surgeon's recommendations," Dr Wright said.

"As was obvious by the looks of fear on the patient's faces at the cancer clinic," she agreed. "It is a fearful situation to be in, I can totally understand people not questioning the recommendations, especially if they don't have any idea that there may be other less drastic options. Anyway, back to the study," she said returning to her report.

"Radiotherapy has been evaluated mainly in trials in which chemotherapy was not given. The widespread use of adjuvant chemotherapy calls for a reassessment of radiotherapy, because the efficacy of systemic therapy in preventing local or regional recurrence after mastectomy is only moderate, and it is not clear whether local or regional control is required for prolonged survival in patients who also receive adjuvant chemotherapy. The aim was to evaluate whether the addition of radiotherapy to total mastectomy with axillary dissection and adjuvant chemotherapy influenced locoregional control of tumors, the likelihood of freedom from distant metastases, and overall survival in high-risk premenopausal patients.

"So here, as I understand it," Ariena said, "they're saying that preventing recurrence by having chemotherapy is not that great, so they wanted to assess if that would improve by having radiation as well."

"Yes," he agreed.

"Right, not very assuring for having chemo then is it? I mean, chemo is also a back-up to having surgery as well," she pointed out.

"Yes, and none of it addresses the cause," he said, "so recurrence is highly likely anyway, if it's the symptoms that are being treated."

\*

"The methods and protocol design used in this study are interesting," she continued.

"The Danish Breast Cancer Cooperative Group protocol includes premenopausal high-risk patients with breast cancer. High-risk status was defined as consisting of one or more of the following: involvement of axillary lymph nodes, a tumor size of more than 5 cm, and invasion of the cancer to skin or pectoral fascia (pathological stage II or III).

"So, the same as me," she commented.

"A woman was considered premenopausal if she had had amenorrhea for less than five years or had had a hysterectomy before the age of 55. To be eligible for the study a woman had to have no evidence of metastatic disease as determined by physical examination, biochemical tests, chest radiography, bone scintigraphy, or bone radiography and no other previous or concomitant malignant disease.

"Same again."

"The study was approved by the national ethics committee, and oral informed consent was mandatory. The departments responsible for systemic treatment and follow-up used a closed-envelope system to randomise eligible patients. No stratification into prognostic subgroups was performed before randomisation. Patients were recruited from November 1982 to December 1989. After surgery, they were randomly assigned to radiotherapy plus cyclophosphamide, methotrexate, and fluorouracil (CMF); CMF alone; or CMF plus tamoxifen.

"There's the methotrexate that was mentioned with the IPT information," Ariena noted.

"Because of a higher than expected rate of mortality, enrollment in the third subgroup was stopped in June1986, as described elsewhere. This report addresses only the results in the first two groups.

"Higher than expected rate of mortality!" she repeated, "so they stopped the third group because most of the people died in the first two groups!" she looked at the doctor aghast. "That tells you right there that this protocol is not successful," she said shaking her head. "I'm thinking that there's every chance it was the treatment, not the cancer that killed them. Of course, the study did not include looking into that!" she added.

"No, it never does," he agreed, "that's because these so-called scientific studies are biased towards the protocol."

"So, when people who are on a study die," she mused, "are they counted in the death-by-cancer percentage?"

"If they still have cancer, yes," he replied.

"...But if the death was caused by the treatment?" she left the question dangling.

"If you have a diagnosis of cancer and you die other than by accidental causes, it's considered that you die of cancer," he affirmed.

"Even if you die during treatment?"

"If a patient dies during treatment it is usually because they suffer cardiac arrest," he said.

"Oh, the primary side effect of chemotherapy," she said nodding, "and the cause of death?"

"Cardiac arrest."

"Not cancer?"

"If cancer is present, it may also be noted."

"That will keep the percentages up," she said, "of death-by-cancer that is." Ariena raised her eyebrows at the doctor. Shaking her head in disbelief, she looked back at the report in her hand. "I'm not liking what I'm reading, but I'll keep going," she said.

"The primary surgical treatment, performed at 79 surgical departments, was total mastectomy and axillary-node dissection.The pectoral fascia was stripped, but neither the major nor the minor pectoral muscles were removed. Axillary dissection included removal of the central axillary lymph nodes involving level I and part of level II. Overall, a median of seven lymph nodes were removed. Grading of anaplasia was performed only in ductal carcinomas. The pathologist recorded the number of lymph nodes identified in the specimen, as well as the gross tumor size and whether there was invasion of the tumor into skin or deep fascia.

"Which with me, there was," she stated, "now, we get a bit technical here, but it's worth the read just to understand exactly what they're talking about when they say radiation therapy, and the depth of the doses.

"In this study, radiation therapy was delivered to the chest wall, including the surgical scar and regional lymph nodes (i.e., supraclavicular, infraclavicular, and axillary nodes as well as internal mammary nodes in the four upper intercostal spaces). The intended dose was a median absorbed dose in the target volume of either 50 Gy, given in 25 fractions over a period of 5 weeks, or

48 Gy, given in 22 fractions over a period of five and a half weeks. The recommended field arrangement involved the use of an anterior photon field against the supraclavicular, infraclavicular, and axillary regions and an anterior electron field against the internal mammary nodes and the chest wall. The use of posterior axillary fields was advised in patients in whom the ratio of the anterior to posterior diameter was too large to limit the maximal absorbed dose to 55 Gy (given in 25 fractions) or 53 Gy (given in 22 fractions). Most of the patients were treated at the six departments that used a linear accelerator, but 64 patients (7.5%) were treated at small departments that used 250-kV x-ray machines. In these patients the minimal intended dose was 36 Gy given in 20 fractions over a period of four weeks. Compliance with radiotherapy was high; only 32 patients (3.8%) did not receive the planned treatment.

"The study that they want me to go on, and say I'm the perfect candidate for, is to determine how strong they can make the radiation before it adversely affects the heart and lungs," Ariena said, "when I said that I wouldn't be doing it, I was given the guilt treatment, telling me that I could be helping so many others if I participate in the study. Again, it's an experiment and people who have had the death sentence are perfect candidates because they're going to die anyway."

"It's the same experiment that's been going on for 40 years," he said, "the only difference in the results would occur if the person in the study was strong enough to endure the treatment, and that won't help others, since everyone has different tolerance levels and, of course, different diagnosis."

"I just can't believe that people don't get it," she said, "I mean, they don't get what's going on. The young radiologist whom I saw was genuinely enthusiastic about the study. She really thought it would be of benefit to others, until I burst her bubble," she added.

"What did you say to her?" he asked, looking at her apprehensively.

"I just pointed out the obvious," she replied with a shake of her head. "Anyway, radiation is not an option in my case, whether they think I'm the perfect candidate or not."

"Well, that's one less thing we have to deal with," he said with a smile, "no mastectomy and no radiation, that just leaves the chemo and hormone treatment."

"Unless we can do some kind of complimentary natural therapy and lower the dose, it's unlikely that I'll agree to those either," she replied, "so let's see what the report says about those." She returned to the file and continued reading.

"For the adjuvant systemic therapy, a combination of cyclophosphamide (600 mg per square meter of body-surface area), methotrexate (40 mg per square meter) and fluorouracil (600 mg per square meter) was given intravenously every four weeks, with the first cycle beginning two to four weeks after surgery. Patients who were randomly assigned to radiotherapy plus CMF started radiotherapy within one week after the first cycle of chemotherapy. They completed the treatment within five weeks and, after a rest of one to two weeks, continued with the CMF regimen, which was repeated every four weeks. Thus, for these patients the planned chemotherapy consisted of eight cycles of CMF, whereas the patients who were assigned to CMF without radiotherapy were given a total of nine cycles of CMF.

"So, without the radiation, there is an extra dose of chemo, interesting how they measure the body surface by square meters!" she commented.

"The patients were followed with clinical examination at regular intervals for up to 10 years and further tested only if they had symptoms or evidence of recurrent disease. All diagnostic, therapeutic, and follow-up data were validated and processed by the Danish Breast Cancer Cooperative Group's data center. The protocol did not call for an interim analysis, but the study was monitored regularly by the data center for excess mortality in either treatment group. To optimize the quality of the data, all events recorded by the data center through June 1992 were cross-checked with hospital records throughout the country to ensure correct recording of the site or sites of the first relapse. Locoregional recurrence was defined as the appearance of local or regional tumor (in the chest wall, axilla, or supraclavicular or infraclavicular area) alone or together with distant metastases (diagnosed within one month after the initial finding of recurrence). Any recurrence that occurred after the first relapse was not included. Disease-free survival was defined as the duration of survival without locoregional recurrence or distant metastases, cancer in the opposite breast, or other malignant disease. Overall survival was calculated as the length of time until death, irrespective of cause. The lengths of time until treatment failure were measured from the date of mastectomy.

"I'm seeing an interesting definition of survival here," she mused, "so while a person has no recurrence they are considered to be surviving disease-free, but when they die, irrespective of the cause (which is not clearly defined at all), it's considered overall survival. Interesting that everyone is considered a survivor even when they die. The other interesting aspect is that treatment failure is clearly expected, since it is mentioned as such, and is measured from the time of mastectomy, the first line of treatment."

"Not only that," he added, "but the study was monitored regularly for excess mortality, do we know what excess mortality is?"

"The study does not address this," Ariena said, "there are no numbers quoted as being considered excess. However it did state earlier that due to excess mortality, the study stopped before taking on a third group of patients. So, that is clearly another 'side effect' that was expected."

"Perhaps when you have a study involving humans," he suggested, "there's a point in the protocol where if the mortality rate from the treatment is excessive, the study is stopped."

"Yes," she agreed, "it wouldn't be good for the results to show that an excessive number of people on the study died, but of course they wouldn't be recorded as dying of the treatment would they, they would have died of cancer. This is definitely becoming a little too insidious for my liking."

"There are certainly many aspects of studies that are far from ideal," the doctor said, "and that's because there are so many variables. Of course the studies conducted by medical protocol are always biased towards proving that the protocol is successful. If the studies included a group of patients who receive complimentary therapy alongside the medical protocol, a group of patients who receive natural or alternative treatment without the medical protocol, and a group who receive no treatment at all, then we would see a much different picture, but of course that will never happen while the studies are funded by the pharmaceutical industry."

"Yes, the results would be much more conclusive," Ariena said, "well, here's what the study says about recurrences.

"The recording of only the first recurrence and not of subsequent recurrences (local, regional, or distant) implies that an estimation of the time to locoregional recurrence would be categorized as an analysis of competing risks. However, the effects of radiotherapy on locoregional recurrence and distant metastases cannot be assessed separately. Any analysis of locoregional recurrence therefore involves analyzing the time to the first recurrence (at any site) and the percentages of patients with locoregional recurrences and distant metastases. The latter are analyzed as simple proportions because the lengths of follow-up and the way censoring was performed in the two groups were similar. These values were compared by chi-square tests and risk ratios. The life-table method was used to estimate the probability of treatment failure for the end points of disease-free survival and overall survival, and the log-rank test was used for comparison.

"Again, it appears that recurrences were expected," Ariena commented.

"A multivariate Cox proportional-hazards analysis was used to evaluate prognostic variables and treatments regarding disease-free survival and overall survival. Statistical analysis was performed by the likelihood-ratio test. Because of the lack of proportionality, the analysis was stratified concerning histopathological findings, ductal, lobular, or medullary carcinoma. Furthermore, the last two histopathological types could not be graded regarding anaplasia, but in the multivariate analysis they were designated as grade I anaplasia. The Cox model was further applied to test whether radiotherapy significantly affected the prognostic variables. Treatment effect was evaluated according to the intention to treat principle, and all the patients were included in their randomisation group irrespective of whether they completed the planned treatment. The evaluation of recurrence and survival and the median potential follow-up was 114 months.

"There's another interesting comment," she noted, "that all the patients were included in the treatment effect evaluation whether they completed the treatment or not. That must mean that some patients did not complete the treatment, so what happened to them? Are they the ones who died or were there some patients who opted out of the treatment part way through?"

"As with all studies, there's a lot alluded to and a lot left unsaid," he replied, "that's usually because those aspects have no relevance to the preferred outcome of the study."

"No relevance!" she exclaimed, "it's not relevant if they die?"

"Not if that is not what the study is trying to prove."

"Right, of course." Ariena took a deep breath and continued reading.

"Of the 1789 patients who underwent randomisation, 81 (34 assigned to radiotherapy plus CMF and 47 assigned to CMF alone) were subsequently found to be ineligible by the data center and were excluded. The reasons for exclusion were the patient's inclusion in another protocol, the occurrence of distant metastases, the presence of other malignant conditions, or the patient's refusal to participate in the study. These patients were included only in the analysis of survival. Of the remaining 1708 premenopausal patients, 852 were randomly assigned to postmastectomy irradiation plus CMF and 856 to CMF alone.

"So, why were the patients that were excluded from the study included in the analysis of survival, to give a better percentage?" she suggested.

"It wouldn't have been to give a worse percentage," he said.

"No," Ariena looked at him, "isn't that fudging the numbers?"

"No comment on that one," he replied, shaking his head.

"Well, the frequency of locoregional recurrences or distant metastases in women treated with radiotherapy and CMF or CMF alone after mastectomy is scary, listen to this.

"By the time of the analysis (median follow-up, 114 months), the disease had recurred in 858 patients and 842 patients had died.

"That means that only 8 people did not have recurrence or die," Ariena said.

"If you go by actual numbers," he agreed, "however, we've already noted that there were some numbers included in the survival analysis that were excluded from the study, so how do we know that these numbers are correct?"

"Exactly, but one thing is for sure," Ariena said, "it states quite categorically that an overwhelming majority of the people included in the study results either had recurrence or died. That makes any other observation or statement regarding the study invalid in my books. This tells me that the protocol used was highly unsuccessful."

"Insofar as the patient mortality and recurrence rate, yes," he agreed, "but that is not what the study was conducted for. The study was to ascertain whether the protocol of radiotherapy combined with chemotherapy was better than chemotherapy treatment alone."

"You're right there," she agreed, "as is shown in the following paragraph." She lifted the file again and continued to read.

"The probability of disease-free survival was significantly higher in the group that received radiotherapy plus CMF than in the group treated only with CMF. The type of first recurrence differed significantly in the two groups. Locoregional recurrence was significantly more frequent in the group treated with CMF alone, whereas distant metastases were more frequent in the group treated with radiotherapy plus CMF. The relative risk of locoregional recurrence as a first event among patients treated with CMF alone was 3.7 (95 percent confidence interval), and the relative risk of distant metastases as a first event was 0.8 (95 percent confidence interval). The estimated overall survival after 10 years was 54 percent (95 percent confidence interval) in the group assigned to radiotherapy plus CMF, as compared with 45 percent (95 percent confidence interval) in the group assigned to CMF alone.

"I notice there is no comment on the fact that metastasis was more frequent in those who had radiotherapy," she said. "Clearly, the radiotherapy either didn't reach the distant metastases or it caused it." Ariena looked back at the paragraph. "There's also not a significant difference in the percentages between both groups," she said, "and I consider the overall survival percentages to be extremely low. It seems like there was a fifty-fifty chance of either having a recurrence or dying. Unless you were one of the mysterious 8 of course."

"Not a good ratio, that's for sure," he agreed, "so, how are the results reported?"

"Results of this study confirmed that tumor size, the number of pathologic nodes, and the grade of anaplasia are the major prognostic factors in breast cancer.

"We knew that already."

"No subgroups could be identified in which the effect of radiotherapy was particularly beneficial.

"Really?"

"It was estimated that locoregional recurrences were the only cause of a first relapse in 80 percent of patients who received only CMF postoperatively, whereas in the group given radiotherapy and CMF, 41 percent of the patients who relapsed with locoregional recurrences also had distant metastases (31 of 75 patients).

"I can't believe that they state the cause of relapse as recurrences," Ariena said.

"I agree with you," he said, "recurrence is a symptom, not a cause. Recurrence is a message from the body saying whatever you are doing is not working. This protocol is to treat the symptoms, not address the cause."

"I was told by the oncologist that they don't know what the cause is, and that they can only treat the symptoms," Ariena said. "When I said that the cure is in eliminating the cause, I was told that there is no cure for cancer. All the so-called research that is being done in the name of finding the cure for cancer is completely useless if they are not looking for the cause."

"Of course they are not interested in finding the cause, or the cure for that matter," he said, it's a multi-billion dollar industry we're dealing with here. There's no profit in making people healthy, but there's huge monetary gain in keeping them sick."

"Yes, and the pharmaceutical industry is keeping up the pretense of looking for a cure, when in reality all those billions of dollars raised every year for research to find a cure, is going into their pockets to keep the industry going."

"The only research that is being done by the pharmaceutical industry is to figure out the maximum dose and strength of their drugs that can be given to humans without appearing to kill them outright."

"The research has been going on for over 30 years and the rate of people with cancer is higher, so anyone can see that their protocols are not working," Ariena said. "When it's so obvious, I don't get why so many people just blindly follow along."

"Because they don't question it," he replied. "The general public have been brainwashed into believing that they can do anything until they get sick, then they have to go to the doctor and get treatment for it. The pharmaceutical and food industries have been marketing that concept for years, and the governments have so-called health care systems in place that offer these protocols and prescription drugs for free, so people don't even think about taking responsibility for their own health. The fast food industry and agribusiness have had a stake in keeping people brainwashed too, people really believe that either what they are eating is good for them, or that nutrition has nothing to do with health."

"I realise that," Ariena said, "but what about the doctors? Surely they must know what's going on?"

"Some do," he said.

"Yes, of course, I realise that too," she said smiling at him. "Well, since we're trying to establish from this study whether to consider the recommended protocol, I'd better read through the rest of this.

"The addition of irradiation to chemotherapy reduced the frequency of locoregional recurrence to about one-fourth that found in the groups that did not receive radiotherapy. The frequency of locoregional recurrences increased with the size of the tumor, the number of positive nodes, and the grade of anaplasia, irrespective of treatment.

"That's contradictory to the previous conclusion," she commented.

"The size of the primary tumor, the frequency and number of positive lymph nodes, the histopathological grade, the use of radiotherapy, and age were all significant independent predictors of outcome and relative risk of any type of recurrence or death or of death from any cause. No significant interactions between radiotherapy and these prognostic signs were found, that is, the beneficial effect of radiotherapy on both disease-free and overall survival applied to all subgroups. Results indicate that the addition of radiotherapy to adjuvant chemotherapy after total mastectomy and axillary dissection reduces locoregional recurrences and improves survival. Previous studies of radiotherapy, which included only small numbers of patients (approximately one-fifth the number enrolled in this study), improve in the control of locoregional tumors and suggested improvement in survival.

"Another contradictory paragraph," she noted, shaking her head.

"Although our protocol carefully described recommendations for the surgical procedure, there might have been important variations in the extent of the surgery performed among the departments that enrolled patients in the study. The surgeons found relatively few lymph nodes in the axilla (median, seven nodes), but the number also relies on the pathologist who counted the lymph nodes in the specimen. The fact that 255 patients had fewer than four nodes removed weakens the analysis of the influence of having more than three positive nodes in the study group. Although the frequency of positive nodes was included in the analysis of prognostic factors, the importance of the number of nodes removed is difficult to assess, since in some patients many nodes were removed because they were clinically involved, whereas in others many nodes were removed by a careful surgeon.

"What do you make of that comment?" Ariena said, raising her eyebrow.

"Perhaps it insinuates that a careful surgeon could remove many nodes whether they were involved or not," he suggested.

"I would hope that all surgeons are careful, or at least capable of doing the surgery," she commented. "The other comment that is interesting is that although the study had a recommended surgical procedure, apparently the surgeons did whatever variations to the recommendations as they saw fit. That's what my surgeon said would be the case when he did the surgery too. So a patient is really in the hands of the surgeon, whether there are recommendations on the study or not."

"Another reason for having a careful surgeon."

"Right," she smiled, "I also find it interesting that the majority of patients had so few nodes involved, however that appears to be in question since there is no way of knowing whether the pathologist can count or not."

"We'll assume that the pathologist was a careful counter then."

"The problem of local recurrence is not related solely to the management of the axilla, since more than half of the recurrences were on the chest wall. Recurrences on the chest wall and in the axilla (without concomitant distant metastases) were treated with curative intent. Most patients who did not receive radiotherapy were treated with resection of the recurrent tumor followed by radiotherapy, whereas patients who had received radiotherapy were treated with surgery alone. The significant difference in overall survival between the group treated with radiotherapy plus CMF and the group given CMF alone indicates that second-line treatment cannot compensate for inadequate primary therapy.

"So, is this saying that the initial surgery was inadequate?" Ariena asked.

"It's very vague, whatever it means," he replied. "What I'm hearing is that the patients who had recurrences had further surgery to remove the recurrent tumour whether they had had radiotherapy initially or not, and those who had not, then received radiotherapy afterwards. I think the comment about inadequacy refers to those patients who did not receive radiotherapy initially," he added.

"OK, interesting choice of words," Ariena said as she looked back at the report.

"The type and dose intensity of adjuvant chemotherapy are also important. The dose intensity with 8 or 9 cycles of CMF (given at four-week intervals) that was used in this trial is lower than the usual course of 12 cycles, a number that was also used in a previous Danish Breast Cancer Cooperative Group trial. This reduction may decrease overall survival, but it is not likely to change our conclusion.

"What? Had they already decided on their conclusion?"

"Perhaps the company who sponsored the study had."

"Right.

"The fact that patients given combined treatment received only eight cycles of CMF, with a long interval between the first and third cycles, might have reduced the benefit of radiotherapy plus CMF. The guidelines for irradiation after mastectomy were based on experience from previous trials, where CMF was given simultaneously with radiotherapy, whereas it was given sequentially in this trial to decrease the early and late reactions in normal tissues.

"I don't get it, were they doing a trial or weren't they?"

"Sounds like they were losing interest at this stage."

"Yeah, I think, so am I."

"Keep going, there's not much left by the look of it."

"Recording of short-term and long-term complications was planned prospectively in all patients, but the data are incomplete, so long-term complications continue to be recorded. Cardiotoxicity was roughly estimated by comparing the survival rates after radiotherapy among patients with cancer of the left breast and those with cancer of the right breast. There is no evidence of a higher rate of death among patients with left-sided tumors, after a median follow-up of almost 10 years. Longer follow-up and more detailed analysis of the actual dose to the heart are needed before final conclusions can be made.

"So, the complications they are talking about are to the heart," she said, "but I don't get why they compared the left and right breast as opposed to the actual survival rate after ten years. Obviously cardiotoxicity is an issue because they don't know the actual dose to the heart or the long term complications. Also, there is no mention of what short term complications are, do you think that is cardiac arrest?"

"Maybe that is what they were hoping to find out through the study that you are considered the perfect candidate for," he suggested.

"I don't think we need to irradiate the heart to know that there will be complications," she replied, "especially if the intention is to give the highest dose possible. Not going there.

"The decentralized randomisation procedure resulted in the enrollment of 81 ineligible patients. However, the inclusion of these patients did not influence overall survival rates (the 10-year actuarial value being 54 percent in the group assigned to radio-therapy plus CMF and 44 percent in the group assigned to CMF alone.

"There it is again, how can they state that by including patients that were excluded from the study, it did not influence overall survival rates?

"Our study strongly indicates that optimal results of the treatment of high-risk breast cancer can be achieved only by controlling both locoregional and systemic tumors. With current surgical methods of treatment, radiotherapy seems required for adequate locoregional control in high-risk premenopausal patients. However, the optimal balance between surgery, radiotherapy, and adjuvant chemotherapy in high risk patients with breast cancer has not yet been found.

"Well, that was a worth while study," Ariena concluded with cynicism. "So the conclusion of this study indicates that current surgical procedures are inadequate, therefore radiotherapy is also required to achieve optimal results in controlling the tumours. The surgeons must have been happy with that result," she mused. "It's also reassuring to note that the optimal balance of the three recommended treatments has not been found," she added with further cynicism. "I wonder where they are looking?"

"Good to see you haven't lost your sense of humour," he said, "cynical as it may be."

"Honestly," she said with exasperation, "that study probably cost millions of dollars."

"No doubt," he agreed.

"I'm almost convinced that they don't have a clue what they are doing," she said.

"It is all an experiment, remember," he replied, "no guarantees."

"Except that your heart *will* be compromised with the radiation and your hair will fall out with the chemo," she said, "oh, and you can get a free wig!"

"Along with the free treatment," he added. "Well, jokes aside," he continued, "what is your overall inclination at this point regarding treatment or therapy?"

"Still definitely no mastectomy and no radiation," she replied with conviction, "as to the chemo, I'll only consider it if I can have complimentary natural therapy at the same time."

"We will find out more about that when I contact my colleague," he said, "but we need to know what the side effects and recommended doses are to establish a protocol."

"Yes, of course," Ariena said, "I have that here in some abstracts of relevant articles as well as some general comments on research into chemotherapy for breast cancer, shall I go through it?"

"Yep, go for it."

"OK, here we go," she said.

"Both total dose and dose intensity of adjuvant chemotherapy are postulated to be important variables in the outcome for patients with operable breast cancer. The Cancer and Leukemia Group B study 8541 examined the effects of adjuvant treatment using conventional-range dose and dose intensity in female patients with stage II (axillary lymph node-positive) breast cancer. Within 6 weeks of surgery (radical mastectomy, modified radical mastectomy, or lumpectomy), 1550 patients with unilateral breast cancer were randomly assigned to one of three treatment arms: high, moderate, or low dose intensity. The patients received cyclophosphamide, doxorubicin, and 5-fluorouracil on day 1 of each chemotherapy cycle, with 5-fluorouracil administration repeated on day 8. The high dose arm had twice the dose intensity and twice the drug dose as the low dose arm. The moderate dose arm had two-thirds the dose intensity as the high dose arm but the same total drug dose. Disease-free survival and overall survival were primary points of the study. At a median follow-up of 9 years, disease-free survival and overall survival for patients on the moderate and high dose arms are superior to the corresponding survival measures for patients on the low dose arm, with no difference in disease-free or overall survival between the moderate and the high dose arms. At 5 years, overall survival is 79% for patients on the high dose arm, 77% for the patients on the moderate dose arm, and 72% for patients on the low dose arm; disease-free survival is 66%, 61%, and 56%, respectively. CONCLUSION: Within the conventional dose range for this chemotherapy regimen, a higher dose is associated with better disease-free survival and overall survival.

\*

"Well, that is not surprising," she commented, "going for the highest dose. The next abstract addresses the side effects of the chemotherapy of a phase III prospective, randomised trial in front-line therapy of metastatic breast cancer.

"This comparative phase III trial of mitoxantrone+vinorelbine (MV) versus fluorouracil + cyclophosphamide + either doxorubicin or epirubicin (FAC/FEC) in the treatment of metastatic breast cancer was conducted to determine whether MV would produce equivalent efficacy, while resulting in an improved tolerance regarding alopecia and nausea/vomiting. The multicentre study recruited and randomised 281 patients with metastatic breast cancer; 280 were evaluable for response survival and toxicity (138 received FAC/FEC, 142 received MV). Patient characteristics were matched in each arm and stratification for prior exposure to adjuvant therapy was made prospectively. The overall response rate was equivalent in the two arms (33.3% for FAC/FEC versus 34.5% for MV), but MV was more effective in patients who had received prior adjuvant therapy, 13%

for FAC/FEC versus 33% for MV, with a better progression-free survival 5 months (range 1-18 months) versus 8 months (range 1-27 months); while FAC/FEC was more effective in previously untreated patients (43%) versus 35%, progression free survival 9 months (range 0-29 months) versus 6 months (range 0-26 months). Toxicity was monitored through the initial six cycles of therapy; febrile neutropenia and delayed haematological recovery was more frequent for MV, while nausea/vomiting of grades 3-4 was greater for FAC/FEC, as was alopecia, cardiotoxicity was the same for the two regimens. MV represents a chemotherapy combination with equivalent efficacy to standard FAC/FEC and improved results for patients who have previously received adjuvant chemotherapy. Toxicity must be balanced to allow for increased haematological suppression and risk of febrile neutropenia with MV compared with a higher risk of subjectively unpleasant side-effects such as nausea/vomiting and alopecia with FAC/FEC.

"Really can't see the point in enduring those side effects for such a short progression-free survival rate," Ariena commented, " I mean, is it worth it to just be surviving, so to speak? What's the point of extending your survival time if it makes you so sick?"

"Good point," he said.

"Especially if you're not sick to start with, which I'm not," she added, "So you have treatment which is supposed to extend your survival rate, but really just gives you another 6 months of sickness. Not making much sense to me.

"Another trial on first-line chemotherapy for women with metastatic breast cancer that compared the efficacy and safety of doxorubicin and paclitaxel (AT) to 5-fluorouracil, doxorubicin, and cyclophosphamide (FAC). A total of 267 women with metastatic breast cancer were randomised to receive either AT doxorubicin 50 mg/m followed 24 hours later by paclitaxel 220 mg/m, or FAC 5-fluorouracil 500 mg/m, doxorubicin 50 mg/m, cyclophosphamide 500 mg/m, each administered every 3 weeks for up to eight cycles. The overall response rates for patients randomised to AT and FAC were 68% and 55%, respectively. Median time to progression and overall survival were significantly longer for AT compared with FAC (time to progression 8.3 months v 6.2 months)]; overall survival 23.3 months v 18.3 months. Grade 3 or 4 neutropenia was more common with AT than with FAC (89% v 65%); however, the incidence of fever and infection was low. Grade 3 or 4 arthralgia and myalgia, peripheral neuropathy, and diarrhea were more common with AT, whereas nausea and vomiting were more common with FAC. The incidence of cardiotoxicity was low in both arms. It was concluded that AT conferred a significant advantage in response rate, time to progression, and overall survival compared with FAC. So in this trial, the patients receiving the lower dose had a better response rate."

"If we use IPT as a complimentary therapy, the chemotherapy dose must be lowered," the doctor said, "but as I said before, the trick will be getting them to agree to it."

"Yes, since it appears that the protocol is to increase the dose or intensity of it," Ariena said. "The following comments on research are interesting, it's all about either increasing the dose, or the density and intensity or the combinations of drugs, not lowering any of it. The other thing is that most of it is directed at patients with metastatic and advanced breast cancer, in other words, those who are not expected to survive anyway.

"Optimising chemotherapy dose density and dose intensity are strategies aimed at improving outcomes in adjuvant therapy for patients with breast cancer. There are, in theory, at least five models allowing the delivery of a higher overall drug dose intensity. These vary according to three main variables: the dose per course, the interval between doses and the total cumulative dose. Cyclophosphamide, anthracyclines and taxanes are among the most active agents for the treatment of breast cancer and, as such, they have been or are currently the focus of prospective, randomised clinical trials testing some of these dose-intensity models in the adjuvant setting. The results of recent trials suggest that anthracyclines, but not cyclophosphamide, are associated with better outcomes if used at higher doses per course and at higher cumulative doses. However, care has to be taken with premenopausal women where an increased dose of anthracycline per course but a reduced cumulative dose appears to produce a worse outcome. Moreover, decreasing the interval between doses, for anthracyclines and cyclophosphamide, does not seem to provide, so far, additional benefits for women with locally advanced breast cancer. This approach is not feasible with docetaxel, since an increase in dose density induces unwanted side-effects. These results represent our current state of knowledge, but clinical trials are being performed to evaluate further the effect of dose intensity, dose density and cumulative dose of key therapeutic agents on patient outcomes.

"It's all such a guessing game," Ariena commented, "there are so many variables with the different drugs and combinations, I find it quite disturbing. It all appears to be a huge experimental program, irrespective of the fact that these are human beings, not just numbers."

"As we've already observed, the primary reason for these trials, or experiments as you rightly name them, is to establish the range of possibilities of the drugs or combinations of them," he said. "Chemotherapy is not, and never will be a cure for cancer, that is because it is so highly toxic to the body. The only way chemotherapy could ever assist in the body healing itself of cancer would be if the drugs were to eliminate only the cancer cells and not affect the rest of the body. It may be possible to achieve that if the dose is lowered to a minimal toxic level and the drugs are directed only at the cancer cells."

"So the idea of using IPT alongside chemo is to create a situation where the cancer cells are grouped together so the chemo only targets them?" Ariena asked.

"Precisely," he agreed. "The cancer cells all gather around the insulin because they are attracted to sugar, so the introduction of IPT into the system just before the introduction of the chemo, makes it easier for the chemo to target the cancer cells en masse so to speak, and the drugs do not range through the body killing other good cells."

"So there's less toxic buildup throughout the body from the chemo as well," she added.

"That's right," he agreed, "and therefore the body is able to start the healing process without having to deal with a huge toxic overload and a lowered immune system."

"Seems to me that if IPT was used alongside chemo, the overall survival rates would be very different," Ariena observed. "Not only that, but maybe the metastasis could be arrested in some patients, the cancer could be reversed if the immune system is not completely shut down by the chemo's toxicity. There would no longer be a need to research how high or dense or intense they can take the dose to. So, why isn't it being done? Why aren't there any trials on this? At least there would be much less harm done."

"I think you just answered your own question," he replied.

"Right," she said nodding, "that could effectively shut down the cancer industry. Imagine if the percentages and rates were reversed, where the majority were recovering, healing and surviving without the toxic after effects."

"With virtually no toxic side effects either," he added, "but then there would be no need for all the other pharmaceutical drugs that are given to suppress the side effects. Well, there's your answer, there wont be any research funded by the pharmaceutical industry that would effectively put them out of business."

"The experimental developments predicted within the industry for the next 10 years certainly back that up," Ariena said, looking back at the report in her hand. "Here's the direction that it is expected to go."

"It is considered that chemotherapy plays an important role in the management of metastatic breast cancer. The anthracyclines (doxorubicin, epirubicin) and the taxanes (paclitaxel, docetaxel) are considered the most active agents for patients with advanced breast cancer. Traditionally, the anthracyclines have been used in combination with cyclophosphamide and 5-fluorouracil (FAC, FEC). The taxanes have single-agent activity similar to older combination chemotherapy treatments. There is great interest in developing anthracycline/taxane combinations. Capecitabine is indicated for patients who progress after anthracycline and taxane therapy. Vinorelbine and gemcitabine have activity in patients with metastatic breast cancer and are commonly used as third and fourth line palliative therapy.

"I'm sorry," Ariena said shaking her head, "but this is ridiculous. What is the point in continuing with third and fourth line chemotherapy? If a patient has metastatic and advanced cancer and they progress after two different rounds of chemo, then isn't it obvious that they are literally prolonging the agony?"

"The experimentation doesn't stop for the comfort or dignity of the patient," he said, "it's designed to prolong the patient's life, therefore it must continue until survival no longer exists."

"Irrespective of whether the patient's life has any quality to it," she added. "I'm not sure how 'novel' you think this is, but here's what is planned for future research.

"Novel cytotoxic therapy strategies include the development of anthracycline, taxane, and oral fluoropyrimidine analogues;

antifolates; topoisomerase I inhibitors, and multidrug resistance inhibitors. A better understanding of the biology of breast cancer is providing novel treatment approaches. Oncogenes and tumor-supressor genes are emerging as important targets for therapy. Trastuzumab, a monoclonal antibody directed against the Her-2/neu protein, has been shown to prolong survival in patients with metastatic breast cancer. Other novel biologic therapies interfere with signal transduction pathways and angiogenesis. The challenge for the next decade will be to integrate these promising agents in the management of metastatic and primary breast cancer.

"That sentence, 'prolong survival in patients with metastatic breast cancer' really sums it up," Ariena said, "it is about prolonging the inevitable, but to what cost?"

"To the patient or monetary?"

"Both," she replied. "Well, the following conclusion regarding a high dose of chemotherapy is absolutely classic, listen to this," she said, continuing to read the final comments.

"In laboratory models of cancer, high dose of cytotoxic chemotherapy correlates with curative therapy, while cumulative dose is associated with longer survival for those who are not cured. These observations suggest a strategy of using high doses when cure is the objective but smaller doses over a prolonged period when palliation and survival are the goal. A strategy combining repetitive cycles of higher doses of cytotoxic therapy, followed by the optimal combination of hormonal and biological agents based on the tumor's receptors might contribute to both the highest possible cure rate and the longest survival. However, the role of high-dose chemotherapy is not well-defined and remains experimental.

"...and will remain experimental while it is so lucrative," she added, "that's really sick."

"It is the sickness industry," he agreed. "Well, apart from what we've already observed, in what direction do you now think we should go for your situation?"

"I'm not agreeing to having chemotherapy unless the dose can be lowered and we can have IPT or other natural complimentary therapy alongside," Ariena stated firmly, "and I'd like to hear your colleague's opinion on the matter before making a final decision."

"I will get in touch with him in the morning and have his opinion for you by tomorrow night," he said, "I'll email you so you can have the information to look over before you come in the following day."

"That's great, thank you," she said, "meanwhile, I'll contact the oncologist tomorrow and put forward the possibility of using IPT as a complimentary therapy alongside their recommended chemo."

"There is every chance she may not have heard of IPT," he said, "but tell her I can fully explain the therapy and protocol to her by phone, and that I would be willing to administer the therapy myself."

"Really?" Ariena said, looking at him with a smile.

"There would not be anyone in the cancer clinic with any knowledge of how to administer IPT alongside chemotherapy," he said.

"No, of course," she agreed, "well I guess that's our next move then."

"Nope," he said smiling, "the next move is to have dinner and then sleep on it." The doctor stood up and helped her to her feet. "I think we've made some great progress here today," he said, "let's hope it will continue that way."

"Thank you so much," Ariena said, "for listening, and discussing, and treating me like a real person, not just another number or statistic."

"You are a very real person Ariena," he said, "and you've taken the first steps to healing yourself by believing in yourself. Doing your own research and understanding the information is paramount in making your own informed choices and decisions. Taking responsibility for, and control of, your own health is the most empowering thing you can do right now. I admire you for that, and I will do everything I can to help you on your journey." He picked up an apple from the basket and handed it to her. "This wont keep me away, but it will keep you going till you get home for dinner," he said with a smile, "I'll work on an immune boosting therapy protocol for you tonight so we can start on that the day after tomorrow when you come in, we might as well let your body know that we're going to be helping out here."

She took the apple. "You really are the most kind doctor I know," she said, "kind, compassionate and very caring, just like a doctor should be."

"Thank you," he said, holding her coat for her as she put it on. "There will be some tough days ahead," he warned her, "but always remember you can email me anytime, and phone me at home in the evenings if you want to."

"Well, again, thank you so much," she replied, "but I hope that wont be necessary, how often will I be coming in for the immune therapy?"

"Every day during the week for the next month," he said, "after that we'll see how you are doing and revise the protocol. It is to be hoped that we'll get it down to three times a week for the following three months, but that will depend on whether you have the chemo or not as well."

"You'll be getting sick of me by then," she said jokingly.

"I hope so," he said, laughing as he held the door open for her.

"Well, I guess you will get used to having me around then," she said smiling at him as she walked through, "because I'm not planning on going anywhere for a very long time. I already told the oncologist that I want a refund on the six months they 'gave me,' but seriously," she continued with a more earnest look, "I don't believe it's my time to die, I truly believe this has manifested as a challenge, and that my recovery, or survival as they call it, will bring to light the options and choices that are available for therapy and recovery, as well as prevention of cancer."

"I'm inclined to agree with you on that," he said smiling, "I'm sure your light will shine for others, and it's certainly preferable if it shines as living proof."

"This was never in any of my plans," she assured him, "but now that I've been thrown in the deep end, and I have you to help me, I'm sure I'll make it." She reached up and gave him an appreciative hug. He returned the hug then held her at arms length, looking seriously into her eyes. "We all have our own plans," he said, "but none of us really know what part we are to play in the big plan, until it is our time. Perhaps this is your time to play your part in the big picture."

"I hope I can figure out what my lines are," she said.

"You will," he replied, "for they've already been written."

She nodded. "Thank you again," she said with feeling.

"Drive carefully, sing all the way home, eat well and sleep well," he instructed.

*

Ariena was just setting the table for dinner when Glen arrived home. "Hi honey, how did it go with Doctor No. Four today?"

"Doctor No. Four as you call him," she said with irritation, "is a Naturopathic Physician."

"Oh, yeah," he said, " how did it go with your Natural-Path?"

"He is a Naturopath," she retorted, still not amused by his

attempt at humour, "a natural path is most likely what I'll be taking."

"OK, I stand corrected," he said, "I was hoping for a smile, did it not go well?"

"Actually, it did go well," she answered, "we went through all the options for treatment, including the possibility of chemo, but it was very draining, so I'm tired and not in the mood for joking about it."

"I'm sorry," he said, putting his arms around her, "it must be very hard on you trying to decide what to do." She leaned into him and felt the comforting warmth of his body calm her. "So, did you decide what you are going to do?" he asked. She pulled away from him and started putting the food on the table before she replied. "Not entirely," she eventually said, "there are still more questions that need answers."

\*

They ate their dinner in silence, neither of them enjoying it very much. Ariena didn't want to go over everything that she'd discussed with the doctor and her husband sensed it. Eventually she stopped eating and pushed her plate away. She could feel her emotions building and was trying not to let them overwhelm her. Then she remembered the doctor's words about how it was better to cry than to hold it in, and she burst into tears.

"Darling, what's wrong?" Glen reached across the table to hold her hand. She pulled her hands away and covered her face as the sobs began to wrack her body. "Oh, sweetheart, I'm so sorry," he said, "I didn't mean to upset you."

"It's not you," she said between sobs, "it's me. There's just so much to research and so many decisions to make, and I really don't know for sure if any decision I make will be the right one."

She wiped the tears away with the back of her hand and tried to compose herself.

"I don't know why you can't just do what the doctors say," Glen said with frustration in his voice, "just have the chemo and radiation and get it over with. All this research is obviously getting you down and is taking up too much precious time, and it's making you confused and upset."

Ariena stared aghast at him. "I can't believe you said that," she said, "how could you even think that? It's not the research that is making me confused and upset, it's you!"

"What do you mean, it's me? What have I done?"

"That's just it, you haven't done anything," she replied, "and you expect me to go ahead with what the doctors say without questioning it?"

"Everyone else does," he retorted, "I don't see why you have to be so different, it works for other people, so why do you think it won't work for you?"

"Just because everyone else blindly follows along, doesn't mean it's the right thing to do," she countered, "and everybody *is* different, which is the very reason why it doesn't make sense for everyone to be having the same protocol. What makes you think that it works for everyone else anyway?" she asked. "The survival rates in the studies don't tell you that."

"I don't care about protocols and studies," he said, raising his voice, "I just want you to have the treatment so we can get on with our lives!"

"Oh, so that's it," she said, "so I'm disrupting our lives now, am I? Just do the treatment so *who* can get on with living, you? There's every chance that my having the treatment will kill me before the cancer does, is that what you want? So you can get on with *your* life?"

"I didn't say that," he shouted, slamming his fist down on the table as he stood up, "you're twisting my words. I just want you to get better, that's what I meant."

"Don't shout at me," Ariena said in a quiet, steady voice, "there's nothing wrong with my hearing. I don't think there's anything wrong with my understanding either. I understand that you want me to get better so we can get on with our lives, but at what cost? Have you even thought about the consequences of my having chemo and radiation? If it doesn't kill me outright, it would make me very sick, there's no question about that. Do you think that is getting on with our lives? Whatever life I may have left, I don't want to spend it being sick and incapacitated. To be honest, I'd rather die and get it over with! Maybe you should just tell me to go to hell and be done with it!"

"Don't say that," Glen said, fear creeping into his voice.

"You have no idea what it's like to be told you are going to die," she said, "and to be told that the only treatment offered will give you another six months of hell before you go. Why would I want to have the extra six months of hell if that's where I'm going anyway?"

"Please, don't say things like that," he pleaded, "I'm just so afraid that if you don't do the treatment that they've recommended, I'll lose you, and I don't want to lose you. I don't want you to die. Please, tell me, what can I do? What do you want from me?"

"I want you to believe in me," she said looking up at him through her tears. "I want your support and love."

Glen stood up and walked around the table, putting his arms around her, he held her close, running his fingers through her hair. "Oh, my love," he murmured, "of course you have my support, and you know I love you. I'm sorry for my outburst, I am just so afraid." Ariena stayed still, savouring the warmth and comfort of being wrapped in his arms. "I know you love me," she said eventually, "and I know you think you are supporting me, but if you are consumed by fear, how can you fully support me?" She pulled away slightly and looked into his eyes. "You think that if I just go ahead with what everyone else does, that I will be okay, but it's not true," she went on. "Perhaps it would be if I believed in it, but I don't. Perhaps that's how it supposedly works for other people, those who survive that is. Maybe they really believe it will help them and it's their belief, not the treatment, that really does the trick."

"Maybe," he said looking at her, "they don't question it."

"That's just it, they don't," she agreed, "but I do. It never made sense to me from the beginning, having treatment that will compromise my body further. My instinct tells me that I need to help my body heal itself. So that's why I must do the research to find out what is best for me. I must take the time now to make sure I have all the information and options so that I can make the right decisions, decisions that I will believe in, and I can't do that if I'm afraid. Fear twists your way of thinking rationally, so I'm trying to let it go, but it's hard if your thoughts are ruled by fear," she added, "so, please, if you really want to support me, you must let go of your fear too," she implored him. He pulled her to him again, kissing her head and enclosing her tightly with his arms. "I will try," he whispered into her hair, "and I will support whatever decisions you make because I know you are putting so much effort and thought into it, and I love you for that. I know you wont give up so easily, I know it's a big struggle for you, but I'm sure you are right, if we can let go of the fear, everything will be clearer. Anyway, we're in this together, right?"

"Yes," she said, "I'd like to think so. I truly believe that it's not my time to die, and not of cancer, but I must get it right and I do need your love and support." He looked deep into her eyes. "I will always love and support you," he said seriously, "no matter what. Just tell me what you need from me and I'll be there for you." He moved his hand to her chin, and tilting her head slightly, he gently kissed her lips. They continued to gaze into each other's eyes, holding the deep connection from within.

"Thank you," she whispered, "for now, that's all I need to know."

*

"Hey Mum, how's it going?" Scott breezed into the room and planted a kiss on his mother's cheek. "Doing some more research?" he asked looking over her shoulder at the computer screen.

"I've just been replying to an email from my Naturopath." Ariena stood up and pushed the chair out, gesturing for him to sit down. "Have a read of his email, while I go and put the kettle on," she said.

"OK, tea sounds good," he added smiling at her. He watched her as she left the room, sighed, and turned to the computer.

> *Dear Ariena, I spoke with my colleague this morning about you and the decisions you are trying to make. He did agree that you do need some kind of chemotherapy because of the aggressive nature of this kind of cancer. The cancer being a high grade makes most of the cells divide rapidly. This makes them more susceptible to the chemo drugs than they otherwise would be. He gave me some very good suggestions for mini-mising immune system side effects and increasing the chemo's effectiveness, which he considered essential if you were to go for the chemo option. It was his feeling that in general patients with this type of cancer had better response with Naturopathi-cally supported chemo than those without chemo. After a long discussion of the pros and cons of chemo he did suggest that in this kind of situation he does try to guide his patients to do the chemo and recommended that I do the same for you whether or not the IPT is available. He is not able to do the IPT. I am*

*not going to talk you into taking chemo but I was encouraged in methods to fully support the immune system while doing chemo. So I feel more confident about seeing a more positive response to chemo. I will be at home this evening, if you would like to talk more please phone me.*

*Remember that if it's not your time yet you are not going anywhere whether you do or don't do the chemo. Maybe the chemo doesn't have to be more scary than it is. I still trust that you can make the best decision for you, not for every other one or statistic with a similar diagnosis, but for you yourself. Try to find the PEACE and resist being pushed either way by fear. Ask God He will give you the wisdom and the PEACE for that matter. Ask and you receive as is commonly said. It is hard to trust something or someone outside of yourself.*

*With my prayers*

Ariena was just pouring the tea when her son walked into the kitchen.

"Well, what do you think?" Scott asked.

"I think I'm extremely fortunate to have such a kind and compassionate doctor supporting me," she replied, sitting down and sipping her tea.

"You're right there," he agreed, "but what about the chemo?"

"I won't do it without the IPT," she replied firmly, "your sister has been doing some research and has come up with the possibility of trials with IPT being done through the Uni. I've mentioned it in my email reply to see if that is a possibility."

"Good idea," he said enthusiastically. She wrapped her hands around her teacup, soaking in the warmth through her hands. "I've also been thinking how fortunate I am to have you and your sister here helping with the research and support," she said, looking at her son. "It really is very comforting to know that I have your support, and of course your dad's," she added with a smile.

"Of course you have our support," he replied, reaching out and taking his mother's hand. "It's been a shock for us all, but it's better to be pro-active and help in any way we can, than to be sitting waiting for the phone to ring."

"Yes, and Mia back home helping with the research too, she has to wait for the phone to ring, have you called her today?"

"I'm going to tonight, that's why I popped in to see if there were any updates."

"Well, I had a long phone call with the oncologist discussing the possibility of having IPT alongside the chemo after receiving the email from the Naturopath," Ariena said, "I wrote all the details of the call in my reply email, you can read that too if you like."

"I will," he said, putting his tea cup down and going back to the computer.

*Hi, Thanks for speaking with your colleague on my behalf. I understand that the aggressive nature of the cancer creates the "What if" factor and that is where my indecision lies. Otherwise, I would have opted for no chemo with or without IPT at the outset, you know that. However, your comment about my not going anywhere if it's not my time yet, is absolutely right. I really don't have any say in the matter, since my fate or destiny is already mapped out and all I have to do is follow the path and be prepared to go the distance.*

*I guess I've done about all the training there is for this and with you as my coach, we should be able to make it to the finish line and win this one. You know I appreciate beyond words what you are doing for me, but as always, thanks.*

*My daughter has been doing more research and suggested that we should talk with the Head of Cancer Research at the*

Uni who is open to discussion with other Naturopaths on any subject and/or case. Apparently there are several clinical trials currently ongoing with naturopathic medicine with and without chemo. There is a possibility that they might be interested in doing trials with IPT. One last attempt?

Meanwhile, here's the latest chapter on "My Life – On Hold".

After receiving your email, I spoke at length with the oncologist this morning. I will give you the basic details of our conversation so you know what has been discussed before you phone her.

I told her that if I was going to have chemotherapy I would want to have IPT and that you have recommended that I have a PET scan done to determine treatment protocol. I asked her what her opinion was regarding the PET scan. She replied that she is the regional expert on the subject and (after explaining how it works), did not think it would be of any further benefit in my case, (nor in most breast cancer cases), as all my other tests and scans have proved to have good results and it would be unlikely that the PET scan would find anything further. There is no funding for it and although she is currently doing a clinical test involving PET scanning, she could not get funding for me to have one done. She did say however, that with her connections, she could get a scan arranged for me as early as this Thursday or next Tuesday, if I decide to go ahead and pay for it.

She said she had read the information I had given her on IPT (the copies you gave me giving the history and explaining how the treatment works) and although she found it interesting, was not convinced as she considered the data to be outdated. I had also given her the IPTQ website to access for further information. She said that she only found four cases of anecdotal evidence of IPT treatment for breast cancer and *that it would appear that there is nothing published nor any clinical trials been done.*

*She also said that she read through everything on the website with a scientific point of view, and found that there was not enough conclusive evidence that IPT was safe and beneficial for her to agree to the protocol of reducing the chemo drugs to one-tenth the dose. She was concerned that with an undocumented treatment her name would be on the line and she would not be willing to agree to any treatment that she was not convinced was in the best interest of her patient. She did say that it was entirely up to me if I wanted to go ahead with IPT, but that she would not reduce the chemo dosage. I mentioned that such a protocol would kill me and she said she certainly did not want to do that. (That's reassuring!)*

*I asked her if she would agree to it if we were to present further documented evidence that IPT is valid and her opinion was that if the Doctors who have been working with IPT for so many years have not done any clinical tests to prove its validity, she would want to know the reason why. She mentioned that if they had been successfully using IPT for over 16 years, they had plenty of time to at least do Stage II tests. She referred to IPT as an alternative treatment rather than a potentiation treatment, even though I have not at any time mentioned naturopathic treatment nor that you are an ND. She said that her recommendation at this point would be to go ahead with the chemotherapy starting treatment next week and have radiation treatment afterwards with possibly hormone therapy (tamoxifen) to follow up. She did say that this is proven and documented and, as she almost (?!) has a degree from Harvard University is in a position to consider herself an expert on the subject. (I did not question the "almost").*

*She agreed to my suggestion that you phone her to discuss the case further, as I had exhausted my knowledge about IPT.*

*She said she is not opposed to learning about any therapy*

*that can potentially help with the treatment of cancer and would be the first to agree to setting up trials if she was convinced it would be beneficial.*

*So, your move.*

*Tomorrow, she will be attending the Cancer Clinic Oncologist's Patient Case Conference and will put forward the idea of IPT for my case, to ascertain if any of the other oncologists have knowledge of it or are interested in its use, and for their opinion whether she should proceed any further with the idea. Of course, she will have a biased opinion if she has not talked to you beforehand.*

*Hope you are able to convince her as well as you have me.*

*Good Luck, Ariena.*

Ariena had been standing behind Scott as he read her email. He looked up at her. "It's tough," he said, "but stay in control Mum, you need to believe in whatever decision you make, so all this research you're doing and discussions you're having will be worth it."

"I know," she agreed, "sometimes I think it would be so easy to just give in to the fear-driven thoughts that are lurking in the back of my mind, but my instinct keeps kicking in and stopping me."

"Thank goodness for that," he replied, standing up and giving her a hug. "By the way, how did the conference call with the other oncologists go," he asked.

"As expected," she replied, "they won't move from protocol, they all agreed with what's been recommended by the oncologists at the Cancer Clinic."

"So, it's back in your court then."

"Yes," she replied smiling at him, "but then, it always has been."

"Isn't that the truth," he agreed. "Thanks for the tea, Mum," he said, kissing his mother on the cheek. "I've got to go now to make that phone call, I'll see you in the morning."

"Say hello to Mia from me, and thanks for your encouragement and support," she replied, "it means so much." Ariena waved as her son walked out the door, a feeling of gratitude bringing a smile to her face.

*

Ariena slowly turned and looked at the phone. For a moment she thought to herself, *how odd it is that I can hear the phone ringing, but I can't see it ringing.* She felt tension mounting inside her as the phone continued to ring, was it fear that was stopping her from answering it? The sheer dread of the message and what consequences it would bring? She continued to stare at the phone after the ringing stopped. She had been expecting the call all morning, *the call from the oncologist that will seal my fate,* she thought. She sighed, then sat down beside the phone and waited. She knew that she had to answer it, get it over with. Her mind had been racing throughout another sleepless night, until finally, in the early hours the options had become clear to her. Either way, she knew what her decision would be.

*

"Ariena, I've had a lengthy discussion with your doctor regarding the IPT treatment that he is recommending," the oncologist said immediately when Ariena answered the phone. Ariena felt her heart miss a beat, then start pounding in her chest. "Yes," she ventured with anticipation.

"Although your doctor is well versed in IPT procedures and appears confident of the possible outcome in using IPT as a complimentary treatment alongside chemotherapy," Dr Price continued, "I am not willing to agree to lowering the dose of the recommended chemotherapy to accommodate the use of IPT. As I mentioned to you previously, without scientific evidence to prove that IPT is beneficial, I cannot allow any deviation from the chemotherapy recommendations that have been made in your case." Ariena said nothing, she waited in silence, hoping that the oncologist might have something else to say, something that might be more positive. "If you wish to go ahead with the IPT, that is your decision," Dr Price stated, "but I will not lower the recommended dose of chemotherapy, so I cannot agree to allowing IPT as a complimentary treatment."

Ariena took a deep breath. "Then, if you refuse to allow IPT as complimentary to a lowered dose of chemo, I will have to decline having the chemotherapy," she said slowly.

"Chemotherapy has been treating cancer for over 30 years," the oncologist replied, "this IPT is not scientifically proven."

"If your decision is final regarding not allowing IPT alongside a lowered dose of chemotherapy, then there is nothing more to discuss," Ariena countered. "I am not going to argue with you doctor, I have done my own research into the matter and am satisfied with my decision. I will not do anything that will compromise my body any further, clearly what I need to do is help my body heal itself. I will therefore proceed with natural therapy to build the immune system."

"Very well, but I must tell you that I do not agree with your decision," the oncologist said. "Since you have also refused to have radiation, I would recommend that at least you should take the hormone medication tamoxifin as prescribed, to lower the oestrogen supply to the cancer cells."

"Thank you for your concern," Ariena said politely, "but I have also been doing some research in that area and since I am at an age where the oestrogen supply could stop at any time through the natural course of menopause, perhaps it is not such a big concern."

"Have you had any symptoms of menopause?"

"I am still menstruating normally, but if you mean hot flashes and headaches, no."

"Menopause can take an extended period of time," Dr Price said, "and I think you are aware that you may not have that much time to wait for the body to take it's natural course, especially if you are not going to have the recommended treatment to slow the cancer down."

"Yes, I do realise that," Ariena replied, "and for that reason, I have been considering another option that would lower the oestrogen levels immediately. Since menopause shuts down the ovaries function of releasing oestrogen and since at my age I no longer need the ovaries to function for reproduction, I could have them removed." Ariena paused, waiting for a comment from the oncologist, but the line remained silent. "I've spoken with my doctor regarding this possibility," she continued, "and I was told that, as my oncologist, your recommendation would be required."

"We have given you our recommendations and you have refused them," came the reply.

"Yes," Ariena agreed, "but I believe that is my right to do so if I wish. I understand that your refusal to agree to my request for using IPT alongside chemotherapy is based on the medical system not recognising IPT as a viable complimentary treatment. However, should I request an alternative treatment or procedure that is available through the medical system, then surely there should be no objection on your part. To be honest," she continued, "I'm not entirely sure that I *will* have the surgery, but I would like the option of discussing the possibility with the gynaecologist, and apparently I need a referral from you to do so."

"That is correct," Dr Price confirmed, "however, in your case, surgical removal of ovaries would be considered electoral surgery and therefore not covered by the medical health care system. If you want to have the surgery, it's up to you, but you will have to pay for it."

Ariena took another deep breath before she replied. "*Surely,*" she said with emphasis, "the medical health care system should be in place for the benefit of the patient, whatever choice they make regarding treatment or therapy. Everyone pays into health care, so everyone should have a choice, but, of course," she continued, "we know it's not set up that way, don't we? Otherwise natural therapy would be available as a choice, wouldn't it?"

"Medical health care is based on scientific proof, natural therapies are not. The government cannot support treatments that are not proven."

"Are you suggesting that chemotherapy, radiation and even surgery is proven to be beneficial to a person's health? Seriously," Ariena replied, "there can't be a doctor or specialist who hasn't questioned it after 30 years of increasing negative results." Without waiting for a reply, she continued, "As I said before, I'm not going to argue with you about the medical system. I will continue to do my own research so that I can make my own informed choices regarding my own health. I have decided not to have chemotherapy and radiation as an informed choice, based not only on my own research but also on the information you have given me. I am now asking you for a referral to the gynaecologist so that I can make an informed decision on whether to have my ovaries removed to lower the oestrogen level. Are you refusing to give me the referral because I have refused your recommended treatment?" There was no reply, only a deafening silence.

"Doctor?"

"If you agree to take the hormone medication, I will agree to write a referral."

"Are you kidding?" Ariena gasped in disbelief. "Even if it worked, I wouldn't need the medication if I have the ovaries removed.

Anyway, tamoxifin is chemotherapy in a pill, and you want me to take it for five years?"

"Tamoxifin has been prescribed for you as a backup to chemotherapy and radiation. If you are refusing to have either, then you must at least take the tamoxifin," the oncologist was speaking in monotone. "The prescription is at the hospital pharmacy in your name, it must be signed for so we will know that you have it. When I have confirmation that you have the prescription, I will send the referral to the gynaecologist."

Ariena shook her head and thought for a few seconds before replying. Finally she said, "I'm not sure that I'm hearing you right doctor, are you refusing me approved treatment?"

Again, there was silence. Ariena waited.

"Pick up the tamoxifin from the hospital and take it as prescribed. The referral you have requested will be sent to the gynaecologist today, you will be contacted for an appointment. Meanwhile, don't come back to us when your natural therapy doesn't work." Ariena felt the slap of rebuke as the line went dead.

*

The door opened and Joy stopped short as she saw her mother sitting in shocked amazement, the phone still in her hand.

"Mum? Are you all right?" She rushed over and gently took the handset and placed it on the cradle. "What's wrong?" The concern in her daughter's voice shook Ariena out of her shocked stupor.

"Sorry, darling," she said, looking up and smiling. "You wont believe what was just said to me."

"You do look shocked, I'll put the kettle on and you can tell me all about it. We'll have it outside so I can watch the car, Kenny's sound asleep."

*

"That's incredible, what a thing to say to a patient. I'm astounded!"

"I know," Ariena replied, "I did expect some resistance to my request for the referral once I'd made my announcement to go with natural therapy instead of their recommendations, but that remark was uncalled for."

"That's bordering on blackmail, not to mention unprofessional," her daughter added, "and to hang up on you, that's not acceptable."

"Good thing I'd been advised what to ask if my request was refused."

"What were you advised to ask?"

"Well, apparently if a medical doctor or specialist refuses approved treatment to a patient, they can be sued and may lose their license to practice. So if you ask them specifically if they are refusing treatment, chances are they will agree to your request."

"Did you say that the record button was on during the conversation?"

"No, but obviously she was not willing to take the risk on refusing the treatment. I think she hung up because she realised that final retort could be damaging to her."

"She obviously wasn't concerned whether it would be damaging to you when she said it."

"Well, I was shocked, but I'm not daunted. I need to stay in control and take responsibility for my own health so I must make my own decisions. I *will not* lose my self respect."

"Atta girl, Mum. Good on you, and we're supporting you all the way. Oh, by the way, this was in the paper this morning and I thought it was interesting. It doesn't quite apply as it's a study about preventing breast cancer rather than treating, but it made me wonder, did they do a genetic test to see if you carry one of the two BC gene mutations? If so, this article seems to indicate that tamoxifen would be helpful if you have BCGA1 gene, but *not* if you have BCGA2. That might help you make the decision about whether to take tamoxifen…"

"Thanks, I'll read it later, but I think I've already decided."

"Sure, but wont hurt to read it anyway," Joy smiled at her mother as she stood to go, "I better go Mum, I think I'm in for an interesting day today, your wee grandson said, 'MINE!' this morning!"

"Oh boy!" Ariena smiled knowingly, "Yep, the fun begins!"

"Anyway, why don't I come with you to see the gynaecologist when you get that appointment."

"Thanks, sweetheart, that would be great," Ariena said, standing to hug her daughter. "I love you."

"I love you too, Mum."

*

"I am surprised that you have a referral from your oncologist considering your diagnosis and treatment recommendations," the gynaecologist commented as he looked up, smiling at Ariena.

"I requested the referral," Ariena replied. "I decided not to have the chemotherapy and radiation treatment that has been recommended, and although it makes sense to lower my oestrogen levels, I would rather not compromise my body further by taking chemotherapy drugs either. So I have been doing my own research into alternative options which is why I'm considering having my ovaries removed. However, I am concerned about having further surgery which is why I wanted a referral to see you."

"I see," he said, smiling at her again. "Well, you needn't worry about the surgery. The procedure only requires day surgery and recovery is very quick."

"Since I already have two beautiful children," Ariena said,

glancing and smiling at her daughter, "I don't suppose I have any need for my ovaries any more."

"Not for reproduction," he agreed. "However, you may experience immediate onset of menopausal symptoms, but those should dissipate within a very short time also. Once removed, the oestrogen level in your body will diminish to almost nil, so the required affect is highly successful." Ariena nodded in agreement and looked again at her daughter.

"It's your decision, Mum."

"I know darling," Ariena replied. She took a deep breath and said, "OK, I'll do it."

"Actually, I'll do it," the gynaecologist contradicted her, "with your permission of course."

Ariena laughed. "Thank you for being so understanding," she replied.

\*

"Hey Mum, how are you doing, are you ready to go?" Ariena put her book into her bag and slipped off the bed. "Yes," she replied, kissing Joy's cheek. "Thanks for coming to pick me up, although I'm sure I could have driven myself home, I really do feel fine."

"We can't leave you to drive yourself home after having surgery, no matter how minor it may have been," Joy said smiling. "Anyway, how was it?"

"Just as he said, very quick and I didn't feel a thing!" she replied.

"Doesn't it hurt to walk?"

"No," Ariena said shaking her head as she walked along the hospital corridor. "There are just two small incisions, with one continuous stitch in each."

"That's great. Do you need to sign out or anything?"

"Yep, at the reception, but I need to go to the pharmacy first."

"What for?"

"I have to pick up my prescription, remember. It was part of the deal."

"Oh, yes, the tamoxifin. You're not seriously going to take it, are you?"

"Figuratively speaking, yes. I'll be taking it out of here." Ariena winked at her daughter as they smiled knowingly at each other.

\*

"You've made my favourite veggie lasagne again, haven't you Mum?" Ariena could smell the unmistakable aroma as she walked through the door.

"You've got to keep your strength up, dear," her mother said as she gave her a hug.

"Don't worry Mum, I'm fine," Ariena replied laughing.

"How did it go, dear?" her father asked, giving her a kiss on the cheek.

"It went well, Dad. Like I said, you don't need to worry, but thank you both for being here."

"Good, then let's eat and celebrate!" her father relied, pulling a chair out for her to sit down. The door opened and Glen came into the room. "Smells delicious in here," he said, kissing Ariena on the head as he sat down beside her, "and you are looking delicious too!" Ariena patted him playfully.

"Surgery went OK?" he asked.

"Yes, no problems there."

"Good, what's in the package?"

"Oh that," Ariena picked up the brown paper bag and took out the tamoxifin.

"So, you really have been given the treatment, haven't you."

"You could say that," she agreed, "yep, you could say that," she repeated with a smile.

# CHAPTER 10

# NATURAL THERAPY

C ome in Ariena," the receptionist beckoned, "make yourself at home." Ariena entered a bright oval-shaped room, with floor to ceiling windows letting in the morning light and affording a tranquil view of the garden outside. There were eight cushioned reclining chairs set around the edge of the room, and the table in the centre had an array of magazines and books, with a small vase of brightly coloured pansies in the middle.

An elderly woman sitting comfortably in one of the chairs, looked up and smiled at Ariena. "Hello, dear," she said cheerfully, "how lovely that you will be joining us."

"Ah, yes," the old man sitting in the chair next to her agreed with a smile, "welcome to the asylum!"

Ariena recognised the couple immediately. "Hello," she said. "I'll be coming every day during the week for a while, so I'm sure we'll see more of each other." She sat down in the chair opposite them. "What did you mean, welcome to the asylum?" she asked.

"Well, that's what we all call it here," the man replied with a laugh, "because apparently we're all just a little crazy!"

"Really? Why do you say that?"

"Well, dear," he said as he lowered his voice conspiringly, "seems like most folks think that we're crazy to shun the medical system, especially when the treatment they offer is free." He turned to his wife and patted her hand. "But we know better, don't we love?" He kissed his wife on her cheek and turned back to Ariena. "My missus was really sick when she was in the hospital, she wasn't getting any better and they said that she wouldn't," he turned back to his wife and patted her hand again. "They said there was nothing more they could do for her and that we should go home to put her things in order. I'm not sure what that is supposed to mean," he said, "but we heard about the good doctor here, and since she's been having this therapy she is getting better every day."

"That's reassuring," Ariena replied, settling herself comfortably into the chair.

"We were coming every day, but now she's so much better, we only have to come twice a week," the old man continued, "and we really look forward to it! It's peaceful here, we can relax in these comfy chairs, read a while or just enjoy looking out at the doctor's beautiful garden."

"Truth be, most of the time, he's asleep," his wife said smiling at him, "but I do feel so much better now, and the doctor is so kind."

"Yep, he sure is that," he concurred, "everyone who comes here says so. One thing I know, it sure beats being in the hospital!"

"Yes, I know what you mean," Ariena agreed.

*

"You're not telling any tall tales now are you?" Dr Wright said, chiding the old man as he entered the room.

"We were just saying to the young lady, that we're all crazy to be here," he retorted with a laugh.

"Well, I'm glad to hear that!" Dr Wright replied, walking over to shake the old man's hand. "And how are you?" he asked the elderly woman, lightly kissing her cheek.

"Better every time I come here," she replied, smiling and patting the doctor's arm, "now don't you take any notice of what he says, we love being here."

"I know," the doctor said returning her smile, "let's get you hooked up." He reached for the mobile stand beside her chair and turned to wheel it towards the counter. "Hello, there," he smiled broadly at Ariena, "welcome to the asylum!" he added with a wink.

"Thank you, I am so happy to be here," she replied.

"

*

While the doctor filled intravenous bags with various fluid solutions, several other patients arrived and settled themselves into the chairs.

"Hello, we have a new inmate!" The old man greeted them all as they arrived. Everyone smiled and greeted Ariena, "Welcome to the..."

"Yes, I know," she laughed, "I'm crazy to be here too!"

The receptionist came in carrying a pot of hot herbal tea and a tray of tea cups. "Lovely to see you all," she said, "who's for a cuppa?"

"What's the flavour today?" a young woman asked.

"Chamomile again, there's so much of it in the garden right now."

"You just want to put us all to sleep!"

"Some of us don't need the tea to put us to sleep!"

"Well, so long as you don't go snoring and disturbing the others."

"We'll give him a nudge if he gets too loud."

Ariena listened to their banter and smiled to herself. She really did feel at home already.

"We all know why he hooked you up last," the old man said after the doctor left the room.

"Really? Why is that?"

"Because you'll be last to finish and you'll get to have a nice long chat with his nibs after we're all gone."

"Oh? Lovely, I'll look forward to it."

"Yes, he likes to explain everything about the therapy he's figured out for you, just so's you know what's going on."

"Good, I like to be well informed, that way I can feel confident with the choices I make for myself."

"You're not as crazy as one might think, then!"

"I think it's good to be a little crazy, adds passion to your life."

"Adds life to your passion, you mean!"

"Yes, that too," she agreed.

"Wait till you get other people's reactions after you've had your therapy!"

"What do you mean?"

"My advice is to go straight home and hide!"

"What? Why would I do that?"

"Don't tell her, she'll find out!"

"Oh, don't listen to them, dear," the elderly woman said coming to her rescue, "they're talking about the smell."

"Smell? What smell?"

"Exactly! You wont smell it, but everyone else will!"

"Please, tell me what you mean, what will everyone smell?"

"Some say it smells like oysters, others say it's like rotten carrots, and there's those who say it smells like rusty iron. Depends on the dose and what you're moving out on the day." "It's the therapy, dear. It is true that you don't usually smell it yourself, but I do sometimes and I get a metallic taste in my mouth sometimes too, but don't worry, it passes."

"Seriously? It passes? You mean, you um, pass gas?" Everyone laughed.

"No, love," the receptionist reassured her as she topped up everyone's tea. "The smell emanates through the pores of your skin as the therapy triggers a detoxing process. It can be quite pungent, but it's only noticeable for about 12 hours, that's why most folks head for home till it dissipates!"

"Oh dear, I was planning to go shopping on my way home today."

"I wouldn't do that, not the first time anyway!"

"You can always act oblivious, how does anyone know where the smell is coming from?"

"I've done that before, I was waiting in the line at the counter one time and the woman in front of me said, 'Can you smell that awful smell?' and I said quite truthfully, 'No, what smell?'"

"I had that happen too, but I said, 'That's funny, last time I was in here people were commenting about a smell, do you think we should be shopping here?'" They all laughed again.

"Is it really that bad?" Ariena asked.

"No, don't be concerned about it dear, you'll get used to it."

"That's easy for you to say," the old man commented, "you're not smelling it!" Ariena raised her eyebrows and looked around the room at the smiling faces.

"Other people can get used to it too, my family don't mind it so much now, they say it's different each time and make guesses what it will be before I get home. It's become kind of a game."

"Is the smell different each time, or people smell it differently to each other?"

"Both, but at different times!"

"We're all different, dear, that's what make life interesting!"

"Wow, can't wait to experience my family's reactions!" Ariena laughed.

"The thing to remember is that it's all natural and it's only doing you good, so most people who do know why there is a smell after you've had therapy are very kind about it and say nothing."

"Yep, kindness and compassion can be just as effective as the therapy," the old man said, patting his wife's hand again.

*

"Looks like you've got about an hour to go before you're all done," Dr Wright said, looking at the intravenous bag. "I've got it dripping slower than usual so we don't overwhelm your system the first time."

"How long would it normally take?"

"Usually 2 to 3 hours at medium drip rate, but it's always better to go slow if we have the time," he explained, "and since we have the time, let's discuss your therapy regime."

"Yes, I was told that we'd be having a nice long chat!" she replied laughing.

"How did you enjoy your first session with everyone?" Dr Wright asked as he returned from saying goodbye to the last of the patients leaving.

"It was rather amusing and quite enlightening, in a good way of course," Ariena replied.

"They can be a little overbearing for the first few times you're here, but they mean well and chatting as a group can be very supportive too."

"Absolutely," she agreed, "I enjoyed their banter, gave me some insight as to each person's character, but overall, it was great to experience the sense of self-worth and hope they all have. I've been reading about all the different natural therapies that I can include to help keep a positive outlook, and laughter is one of them."

"That's why there's no such thing as a bad laugh," the doctor commented as he reached for her file. "Positive emotional states such as love and laughter have a powerful influence over the body and boost the immune response. You know, keeping your sense of humour and maintaining a positive mental attitude has been an empowering strategy for you," he continued, "and becoming proactive by researching alternative options has also given you a firm sense of control. These, together with a strong sense of hope, will profoundly aid in your healing process."

"Yes, I believe you are absolutely right," Ariena agreed, "I feel so different now than I did when I first got the diagnosis, I was almost engulfed with fear then. Now I think of the cancer diagnosis as a gift, an opportunity to transform my own life and perhaps help others by sharing my experience."

\*

Dr Wright looked at her and smiled. "I understand how you will be feeling passionate about sharing your experience and knowledge gained from it," he said, "but right now the reality is that you need to focus on caring for yourself. Sharing with others can come later."

"I suppose you're right again," she replied smiling at him, "I just think everyone should know what their options are and where they can get the right information, so they can make their own informed choices, instead of blindly agreeing through fear."

"Everyone has the power to control their own thoughts and create their own reality," he countered, "when the time is right, they will know."

"But, how will they know if they are not told, not given other options?"

"I'm sure you will be able to help and inform others in the future, but as I said, right now you must focus on you. First you help yourself, then you will be able to help others."

"That is so true," Ariena agreed, "it's similar to what my grandmother always said; how can you love others if you do not love yourself first?"

"Indeed, and loving yourself is the first step to healing yourself.

The most efficient healer of the human body is the healer within, your body's own immune system. So with much love, and help from the natural therapies and treatments that I'm recommending for your regime, let the healing process begin!" he said, placing the open file on the table with a flourish.

"Love a bit of drama!" Ariena laughed. "So what's the plan of action?"

\*

"First, and foremost," he began, "all our therapies and treatments are based on the natural approach of doing no harm. You will not have any negative side effects, only positive responses. However, the body may respond to any therapy or treatment by releasing toxins into the blood stream and thereafter eliminating them through the natural process. This may cause some discomfort, but it will pass once the toxins are eliminated. You do not need any medication for this, rather, we will monitor the response and regulate the treatment or therapy accordingly to keep any discomfort to a minimum. That way we know what is happening and we're not masking symptoms or messages from the body with other medication."

"Sounds good," Ariena said, "and makes perfect sense."

"As it should," he agreed.

"I'm thinking you will have some nutritional advice as well?"

"Oh, yes," the doctor said, "we've all heard the old saying, you are what you eat, well, nothing could be more true. The body has a response to everything you eat, and since you are the one in control of what you put in your mouth, it's entirely up to you to make sure whatever you eat and drink will have a positive affect on your health."

"I've been vegetarian most of my life and never eat any junk food, so I was shocked at first when I got the diagnosis," Ariena mused, "I thought I had a healthy diet, but there's more to it than the food isn't there?"

"Exactly," he replied, "the food plays a big part, but every lifestyle choice we make has a role in achieving optimal health. It's a well balanced wholistic approach that will make the difference, but we'll go into the nutritional aspect in more detail when you come tomorrow."

"So what is in the intravenous drip?" Ariena asked.

"Considering your diagnosis and prognosis, and of course the research you have done regarding the cause in your case," he replied, "clearly we need to reverse the progress of the cancer by giving the body the help it needs to rebuild and rejuvenate the immune system. We also need to eliminate the toxic buildup and ensure that you are not exposed to and can continue to eliminate any further toxic substances," he added. "Accordingly, I have established a protocol of natural immunotherapy, a combination of natural substances to enhance the body's immune system, chelation therapy which removes heavy metal toxins from the body, and ozone treatment, which helps strengthen the immune system, all of which are administered intravenously."

"So that's what I'll be having when I come here," Ariena said, "meanwhile is there anything I can be doing to compliment these therapies?"

"Yes, there most certainly is," he replied, "the therapies are designed to help boost the immune system and therefore the healing process. However, our main aim is to, dare I say the word, *cure* the immediate problem, so you can go on to lead a long and healthy life. You will need to take into account every aspect of your past and existing lifestyle and decide what choices and changes you can make to continue improving your health."

"I can do more research while I'm here, but I'm sure you have plenty of suggestions?"

"I do," he agreed with a smile, "and we can go through some of them as I explain the therapies, since they are all interconnected. There are many lifestyle choices for you to be aware of and possible changes that you can make that will not only compliment the therapies, but can be incorporated in your everyday life. After all, you are about to embark on the adventure of your life!"

"Well put," she nodded, "and I *will* treat it that way. So, go ahead and tell me what to do doctor!"

\*

"Back to your question, what is in the drip, the combination of ingredients in the immunotherapy may vary each day," he explained, "but it will include vitamins, minerals, and some herbal and other plant based nutrients that are known to enhance the immune system. I will explain about each ingredient as I introduce it, but for instance we will be including vitamin B17, which selectively targets and destroys cancer cells while healthy cells remain unharmed. The substance is naturally occurring in many plant foods, including apple seeds, bitter almonds and apricot kernels, which you can also include in your diet. This important vitamin, also known as Laetrile, has four decades worth of clinical evidence and case studies to attest to its efficacy."

"That's interesting, I was just reading about that yesterday," Ariena said, "it was in my mother's collection of health books. She has always said we should eat the whole apple, seeds and all, and she has always eaten almonds and apricot pits every day."

"The first person you should always listen to is your mother," the doctor said, "they always know best."

"Right again," Ariena agreed, "my mother said after she read about Vitamin B17, she immediately included the almonds and apricot pits in her diet to prevent cancer, so she gave me the book to read and said it should work if you have cancer too."

"Great reasoning, you're lucky to have a mother who takes the time to research about health, and who cares enough to share the information and act on it herself."

"Yes, she is a gem," Ariena agreed with a smile, "her whole life revolves around her family and our health. I am blessed to have her."

"Indeed," he agreed, "now, to ensure that the regime is balanced, the combination of immunotherapy, chelation and ozone treatment will vary throughout the week." He reached over to the intravenous bag and adjusted the drip valve. "Not much to go," he said, pouring a glass of water and handing it to Ariena. "Sip this while I explain about the immune system first," he said, "now, as you know, the immune system protects the body from infectious organisms, and it works with the body's other cells and tissues to maintain stability and balance, and overall good health," he continued. "The immune system is our body's natural defense against harmful substances *and* it monitors the body's internal environment for abnormal cell development. There are various groups of white blood cells that possess an innate intelligence for healing. They identify, attack, destroy, and finally remove abnormal cells through the body's lymph system and organs of elimination. Any cell within the body can mutate in response to negative stressors, but a healthy immune system will stop its growth and defend against an uncontrollable malignancy."

"How do the cells mutate and become cancerous?"

"Well, every day an adult produces some 300 billion new cells. They usually divide as they should, but sometimes, chemical or physical agents can sabotage and rearrange the genes that regulate normal cell growth and differentiation. When this occurs, that single cell may begin to divide uncontrollably, multiplying and joining to form a colony of mutant cells," he explained, "but when a body cell becomes cancerous, its membrane may change slightly, so that it bears markers somewhat different from the body's own."

"So, what happens then?"

"Ordinarily, the immune system will recognise and react to the new markers, eliminating the mutant cell," he continued, "but a cancer cell may shed its antigen markers or camouflage itself behind a coat of protein resulting in the system failing to react. At such times, a single mutant cell may escape detection, divide and multiply and form a malignant tumor that invades and destroys surrounding healthy tissue."

"So I guess my cells were sabotaged by the overload of toxins I was exposed to, which would have also prevented the immune system from detecting and destroying them." "Most likely," he agreed, "however, the immune system is also subject to the perpetual cycles of change within the body. For instance, a deficiency of essential nutrients, stress, or even dietary excess can also affect the immune system function. Nerve cells and immune cells are interconnected and there is a complex connection between the immune system and the brain. Some immune cells have receptors on their membranes for chemicals produced by the brain. One group, known as endorphins, may at times reduce our resistance to dis-ease in the body. Endorphins produced in response to mental stress, both moderate and severe, can suppress the activity of T-cells which are the elements that make up the body's defences."

"Don't endorphins have the reverse effect during exercise?" Ariena commented.

"Yes, most definitely," the doctor replied, "the exhilaration and overall feeling of well-being experienced during and after exercise is produced by endorphins boosting your immune response. Therefore, regular exercise is an important factor in boosting your immune system."

"Well, I can take care of that side of things," she replied smiling, "I go for a run almost every day, so I'll just have to increase the distance I suppose."

"You certainly can, but remember to keep within the limits of your capability," he reminded her, "just make sure you don't increase too much, too soon or too fast."

"Yes, I'm well aware of that," Ariena agreed, "that is the cause of most injuries."

"In your case, we must be aware that your immune system will be working hard on the healing process, so endorphins produced in response to overexertion can also suppress the body's defences," he warned, "it's a matter of keeping everything in balance, and using strategies to strengthen and build these natural defences to eliminate the cancer."

"OK, I promise to keep the speed down on the corners," Ariena said with a laugh.

The young doctor smiled. "Regular exercise speeds up the elimination of toxins and is necessary to keep the body oxygenated and improve lymphatic function while building immunity," he said, "but any form of regular aerobic exercise, 3 to 4 times a week for at least 30 minutes, will reduce stress and benefit the immune system, it doesn't have to be running."

"I know, of course you're right," she agreed, "but running gives me the freedom I need from the stress of all this, and I can meditate and go within while I'm running. Mostly I love it because it makes me feel alive!"

Dr Wright smiled at Ariena's passion. "Well, that's what we want," he said, "but there are several other factors that play a key role in ensuring optimal immune system function. Most of these I know you are already aware of, but we'll go through them so you can actively identify and implement each factor that may positively affect your health." He handed Ariena a pen and note-pad. "Here, make a few notes so you can do more research on these factors."

"Thanks, nothing like being pro-active!"

"Exactly," he replied.

*

"As I explained before, you need to identify and eliminate all toxic elements from your environment. Removal of accumulated toxins and metabolic wastes is required for effective healing and you also need to consciously avoid any further toxic exposure and environmental toxins that will inhibit the healing process. Toxic chemicals found in cleaning agents and cosmetics, along with pesticides and chemicals used in non-organic farming are poison-ous to the body. All synthetic food additives such as preservatives, colouring and fillers are harmful to the body. Make sure you read the labels."

"I don't use any food additives or cosmetics, and I usually use vinegar or lemon juice for cleaning, but I'll check all the products I have and get rid of anything that is suspect."

"Good. Avoid any synthetic remedies, antibiotics and addictive drugs of all kinds. Suppressing the symptoms with medication is counterproductive because most drugs also suppress the immune system, and of course, addictive drugs create instabil-ity and imbalance within the body, which again, compromises the immune system."

"I've never taken any drugs or medication apart from what was given to me for surgery, and I certainly wont be starting now!"

"I'm sure," he replied, "but as you know, there are man-made chemicals and toxins in the air we breathe, in the unsuitable food we eat and drink, and in cleaning and beauty aids we handle and rub into our skin."

"Like the harmful toxins that I was exposed to," Ariena added.

"Yes, paint and nuclear fallout are so foreign to the body that the immune system cannot flush them out, so they built up causing distress and eventually cell mutation."

"That is why having the conventional treatment of cancer with the use of chemical therapy just doesn't make sense," Ariena mused, "not only is it known to destroy the immune system, but adding such highly toxic chemicals to the body's already compromised system must put it further into toxic overload."

"So many patients go through chemotherapy with that result," the doctor agreed, "and then, often as a last resort, turn to natural therapies to rebuild the immune system. Unfortunately in some cases, the chemical therapy renders the body incapable of future response to nutritional or immune-boosting approaches to cancer treatment."

"I'm so glad we did the research and explored all the options so I could make an informed decision not to have chemotherapy," Ariena said, "at least my body wont have to deal with the after effects of that as well."

"Exactly," he agreed, "everything we do will be a positive move towards healing. The body, through its resilience, will heal itself when given what it needs."

"There are various practices and lifestyle changes that will also help purify the body that you can implement immediately," the doctor continued, "for instance, rebounding on a mini-trampoline to move lymph fluid, flush waste, and increase the number and activity of white blood cells should be part of your daily regime."

"Any particular mini-tramp you recommend?"

"You don't have to buy one if you don't have one, just sit on the edge of the bed when you wake up in the morning, and bounce gently for 5 minutes, that's all it takes to get the lymphatic system working."

"Great, I can do that!"

"If you have access to an infrared sauna," he continued, "a half hour per day exposure to far infrared rays will help to move heavy metals from the body while you are relaxing."

"What's the difference between an infrared sauna and a regular sauna?"

"Well, when your body is exposed to highly toxic substances that it cannot immediately remove, such as heavy metals and chemicals, it stores them in the water molecules of the body to keep you safe. However, if you continue to be exposed, whether environmentally or through lifestyle practices, including what you eat, then those toxins build up in the body and eventually, over time, you have a toxic overload. As you know, this causes dis-ease and imbalance which can lead to cancer," he explained, "so, it is essential to continually lower the toxic levels in the body. Now, back in our grandparent's day, that was easily achieved by being in the sun every day while they tended to their garden or ploughed the fields. Far infrared rays are the beneficial rays of the sun, they have a vibrational affect on the body which releases toxins and eliminates them through the natural process. However, our grandparents were not exposed to so many toxic substances as we are today. Most of the chemicals, pesticides and pollution that we are exposed to today have come into existence since the industrial revolution and both world wars. It is due to the pollution that we've created, that we can no longer be in the sun all day."

"Yes, we are our own worst enemy aren't we?" Ariena commented.

"In some ways yes, but hopefully we will continue to develop ways to counteract some of our mistakes," he said, "as we have with the far infrared sauna. About 30 years ago, the technology of using these rays was researched for use in hospitals in Japan. The technology has since evolved to conducting the far infrared rays through carbon in a sauna application and is now used in health spas throughout the world. The vibrational effect works exactly as if you were exposed to the sun, and the heat causes perspiring which purges toxins through the skin and has a relaxing effect, so the benefits of using an infrared sauna are threefold."

"So it's the warmth *and* the infrared rays of the sun that make us feel so relaxed when we're in the sun," Ariena said.

"Yes, and we also emit and receive infrared rays ourselves, you know how you feel when someone smiles or when you hug someone," he said, "that warm and fuzzy feeling is created by our own infrared rays."

"You're right, we just don't give it any thought," Ariena said smiling, "so, more smiles and hugs, then. Do you know if there are there any local spas that have infrared saunas?"

"Not that I know of," he replied, "but if you do the research on availability and let me know, I'll consider putting one in here."

"I'm on to it," Ariena replied enthusiastically.

"Good," he said as he checked the drip again, "looks like you'll be done in about 15 minutes. Now, with all these ways of detoxing your body, there is a potential for what we call a healing crisis to occur," he continued, "that means you may experience symptoms that are uncomfortable due to having toxins released into the body's system, but there are several ways to help with the elimination of released toxins. One is to drink plenty of water to help flush the toxins through. Toxic buildup can also be released through fasting, which helps to heal and rejuvenate the body. I'll tell you more about fasting tomorrow when we discuss your nutritional requirements."

"Yes, that was something I wanted to discuss," Ariena commented, "I've also heard that juice fasting is a good idea to start with."

"It certainly is," he agreed, "juice fasting keeps your nutritional levels high while allowing the body to rest from digesting solid foods. Juicing also alkalizes and cleanses the tissues, so it's an essential component in the healing process. It is also beneficial to begin a healing regimen with a cleanse to the organs of elimination, the kidneys, liver and colon, which will help remove stored toxins. We'll go more into that tomorrow too," he added.

"From what I've been reading, it seems like there is a wide range of healing regimes established by different doctors and holistic practitioners over the past fifty or so years," Ariena said, "are there any in particular that you would recommend including in my regime?"

"I'm sure they all have their merits," he replied positively, "however, I recommend you research them well and we can discuss any that you are interested in. It is important that we keep the overall regime in balance. There most certainly will be some aspects that we can include, for instance you may already have heard of the Breuss Cancer Cure and the Gerson Therapy, both I would recommend looking into."

"I have come across them, but haven't studied all the aspects yet," Ariena replied. "Aren't they based on juicing?"

"Yes, along with other practices that can also be considered, such as using castor oil packs to enhance circulation, stimulate the immune system and aid in detoxification, as well as using coffee enemas to prevent the reabsorption of toxins."

"I'm not sure I want to put coffee in my body, I don't even drink it!"

"I'm sure your adrenals are thanking you for that," he laughed, "but using coffee enemas cleanse the blood and liver, and counteract the symptoms of a potential healing crisis, quite different to drinking it!"

"OK, I'll read up more about it," Ariena said, "what about the Breuss Cancer Cure?"

"It's based on a very specific juice fast, I have a copy here you can take with you." He stood up and walked over to the bookshelf. "Here it is," he said. He hand her a small book. "Your drip is finally finished," he said, gently extracting the needle from her hand, "shall we go out into the garden and have some herbal tea while we go over a few more things? I don't want you driving just yet, best to wait a half hour or so."

"Oh, that would be lovely," Ariena replied. "You go on out and I'll bring the tea in a minute when I've cleaned things up here."

Ariena stepped outside and took a deep breath of fresh air. She walked over to the garden seat set amongst rows of pansies and sat down. The seat faced west, overlooking a field lush with green grass. A few sheep grazed peacefully with their heads down and tails twitching. Ariena smiled at the thoughts that came into her mind of 'flowers all in a row' and 'tails wagging behind them'. She gazed out at the tranquil scene, feeling the warmth of the setting sun on her face.

"Taking in some infrared rays I see," Dr Wright commented cheerfully as he handed her a cup of sweet-smelling herbal tea.

"Mmm," Ariena replied, "the sun does make you feel warm and fuzzy."

"It's an easy thing to incorporate every day," he said sitting down beside her, "sunrise and sunset, the best times of the day, and most importantly, it will also help you to relax and control any stress." He sipped his tea and looked towards the setting sun.

"Stress increases adrenal hormones that stop the formation of immune cells and overtax your immune response," he continued, "to help relieve stress, you should also continue to practice meditation and yoga whenever you can."

"Like while I'm here?" Ariena said, "I do yoga at home everyday, but I could meditate while I'm in the chair here."

"Absolutely," he agreed, "and, since you already meditate sometimes while running, you could also plan to stop somewhere on the run and meditate. Choose a peaceful spot in the forest or on the beach, somewhere with natural surroundings."

"Yes, I love to run in nature, so I will make the time to include a meditation break while I'm out there," Ariena agreed, "I also like to do my stretching, to release any acids from tissues after running, and other exercises, including conscious breathing, while I'm outside, whether in sunshine, rain or snow!"

"That's great, plenty of fresh air and sunshine is what every good doctor recommends. Speaking of sunshine," he continued, "vitamin D from sunlight has been shown to shrink tumors, and research now links the lack of sunlight to certain cancers. Obviously, you should avoid overexposure during the hottest part of the day, as sunburns can damage skin and promote cancer."

"I can just imagine bringing the drips outside in the garden on a sunny day," Ariena laughed.

"You can always come out here for a while before you go home, and you could also come early to sit in the garden before your therapy," he suggested.

"I might do that, but you might find that everyone will follow suit and you'll arrive to find us all in the garden," she warned, "and some of us might be so relaxed we'll be asleep!"

"That wont do any harm at all," he smiled, "getting plenty of restful sleep is also a very important part of an effective healing strategy. The value of adequate sleep should not be overlooked because without it, our healing efforts will be compromised. It's while you are asleep that the body releases potent immune enhancing compounds, which help to rejuvenate, detoxify, and regenerate the entire system. The liver works to break down and eliminate carcinogens during the deepest level of sleep. Additionally, sleeping in complete darkness contributes to healthy levels of melatonin, which is a hormone secreted by the pineal gland, that cuts off the blood supply to tumors and promotes restful sleep. So a nap in the garden is restful, but you must be conscious of getting enough sleep during the night, at least eight hours or more is required for the body to do it's job."

"I've heard that the most important hours of sleep are those before midnight."

"That's correct, the old saying of early to bed, early to rise, means more than most people might realise. Also, it's important to practice eating the last meal of the day at least three hours before sleep, so that the digestion process will not interrupt the body's healing efforts during sleep. So, we'd better quickly go over the other intravenous therapy and treatment you'll be having, so you can get home for dinner and an early night," he added. Ariena picked up the notepad she had brought with her and sat poised with her pen. "I'm ready for more info."

"OK. Chelation therapy is the administration of chelating agents to remove heavy metals from the body," he began, "it has a long history of use in clinical toxicology. Poison centres around the world are using this form of metal detoxification. To give you a bit of it's history," he continued, "chelating agents were introduced into medicine as a result of the use of poison gas in World War 1. The first widely used chelating agent, the organic dithiol compound dimercaprol, was used as an antidote to the arsenic-based poison gas. The sulphur atoms strongly bonded to the arsenic, forming a water-soluble compound that entered the bloodstream, allowing it to be removed from the body by the kidneys and liver, but," he added, "it had severe side-effects.

"Then, after World War II," he continued, "because a large number of navy personnel suffered from lead poisoning as a result of their jobs repainting the hulls of ships, the medical use of EDTA (ethylenediaminetetraacetic acid) as a lead chelating agent was introduced. Unlike dimercaprol, it is a synthetic amino acid and contains no mercaptans, so EDTA side effects were not considered as severe. It was not until the 1960s that DMSA, (dimercaptosuccinic acid), a related dithiol with far fewer side effects, replaced both the previous agents, becoming the US standard of care for the treatment of lead, arsenic, and mercury poisoning, which it remains today. For the most common forms of heavy metal intoxication, those involving lead, arsenic or mercury, a number of chelating agents have also since been discovered and are available. They all function by making several chemical bonds with metal ions, thus rendering them much less chemically reactive, the resulting complex is water-soluble, allowing it to enter the bloodstream and be excreted harmlessly," he explained, "and since DMSA has been most recommended, we will be using it in the intravenous protocol for your chelation therapy."

"So, it's the DMSA that gives off the metallic smell everyone was talking about," Ariena said.

"Yes, that's it," he confirmed, "but you don't have the chelation every day, like you do the immunotherapy."

"Oh, good, so I'll get a break from comments then."

"Your family and friends get used to it," he said, "and you wont smell it at all."

"Yes, that's what I heard, still if that's the only side effect, it's nothing to worry about."

"Exactly," he agreed, "but I'm sure you'll enjoy the side effect of the ozone treatment."

"Really? How so?"

He gave her a knowing smile and continued. "Ozone therapy

may be administered in a variety of ways," he said, "it may be used therapeutically in the home by drinking ozonated water and using ozone saunas. However we will be using autohemotherapy, a method of administering intravenous ozone infusions (commonly called ozone treatment), by removing between 10-15 ml of your own blood, passing it through an ozonating machine which infuses the blood with a mixture of oxygen and ozone, then reinjecting it back into your bloodstream."

Ariena raised her eyebrows. "Isn't that more commonly called blood doping?" she asked.

"In sporting circles, yes," he confirmed, "It has been known to be illegally used to enhance an athlete's performance."

"So, I'll notice a difference if I were to go for a run after having ozone treatment?"

"Possibly," he said with a smile, "but that's not it's purpose here. You see, the more toxic the body, the less oxygen is delivered to the cells, and oxygen starvation at the cellular level leads to disease in the body," he explained, "however, cancer cells cease to grow when blood and tissues are sufficiently oxygenated. The rationale behind bio-oxidative therapies, as oxygen or ozone therapy is sometimes known," the doctor continued, "is the notion that as long as the body's needs for antioxidants are met, the use of certain oxidative substances will stimulate the movement of oxygen atoms from the bloodstream to the cells. With higher levels of oxygen in the tissues, bacteria and viruses are killed along with defective tissue cells, the healthy cells survive and multiply more rapidly, and the result is a stronger immune system."

"Makes sense again," Ariena commented.

"Yes," he agreed, "and apart from improving the delivery of oxygen from the blood stream to the tissues of the body, there are numerous other benefits to ozone therapy. For instance, it increases the efficiency of antioxidant enzymes, increases the flexibility and efficiency of the membranes of red blood cells and stimulates white blood cell production, thereby helping the body to fight infections and cancers. It also speeds up the breakdown of petrochemicals and speeds up the citric acid cycle, which in turn stimulates the body's basic metabolism."

"Wow," exclaimed Ariena, "I guess it's all that stimulating and speeding up that enhances performance with the athletes, this could be fun!" He smiled at her enthusiasm. "So, what is ozone, and is the treatment safe?"

"Good question," he replied, "ozone itself is a form of activated oxygen, O3, produced when ultraviolet light or an electric spark passes through air or oxygen. It is a toxic gas that creates free radicals, the opposite of what antioxidant vitamins do. Oxidation, however, is good when it occurs in harmful foreign organisms that have invaded the body, and ozone inactivates many harmful bacteria and viruses."

"How long has it been used therapeutically?"

"Ozone has been used since 1856 to disinfect operating rooms in European hospitals, and since 1860 to purify the water supplies of several large German cities," he replied, "however, it was not used to treat patients until 1915, when a German doctor began using it to treat skin diseases. During World War I, the German Army used ozone to treat wounds and anaerobic infections. It was in the 1950s, that several German physicians used ozone to treat cancer alongside mainstream therapeutic methods. It is estimated that as of the late 1990s, about 8,000 practitioners in Germany were using ozone in their practices, and that includes medical doctors as well as naturopaths and homeopaths."

"Sounds good, bring it on," Ariena said.

"Again, we wont be doing the ozone treatment every day," the doctor replied, "but I'll let you know the day before so you can prepare to go for a run afterwards if you like."

"If you think it will be okay," she replied questioningly.

"Oh, yes, the amount of ozone we'll be using is nothing like what has been used in blood doping," he assured her, "but I think you will feel a slight difference in your speed and running style."

"What do you mean, how will it change my running style?"

"You may feel like you're not touching the ground!"

"Really? Okay, definitely bring it on!" she laughed.

"Of course, there are other ways to oxygenate the body other than regular exercise," he replied, "such as deep conscious breathing and adequate consumption of pure oxygenated water. Of course the obvious simple method to increase oxygen intake is by including a highly alkaline diet, preferably at least 80% of the food eaten raw. This raises the body's internal pH which enhances the transport of oxygen to the cells."

The doctor stood up and held out his hand to Ariena. "It's time for you to be getting off home," he said kindly.

"You too," Ariena said, smiling as she took his hand and began walking companionably beside him, "thank you so much for taking the time to explain everything."

"It's all part of the deal," he replied, returning her smile, "I am more than happy to give you all the information I can so that together with the knowledge you gain from your own research, you can make your own informed choices, but, as you know, all the knowledge in the world is of no use to you unless you act on it. Knowledge requires action to achieve results, and that part is entirely up to you."

"Yes, I know," she agreed, "and I plan to do just that. I've promised myself that I'll do 100 per cent the best I can in everything, that way I should get 100 per cent positive results. I'm sure the more I learn, the more I'll incorporate in my lifestyle, I'm getting quite excited about it!"

"Well, that's a good sign," the doctor nodded, "keeping your spirits up and being passionate about what you are doing, no matter what it is, always has a positive affect on your health."

*

Dr Wright opened the door and stepped aside for her to walk in.

"Mmm, it's warm in here," Ariena said appreciatively, "I didn't notice it was getting cooler out there, I was so absorbed in everything you were telling me."

"Yes, it gets cool quickly when the sun starts to set," he agreed as he held her jacket for her to put on.

"Thank you for suggesting we go out in the garden," Ariena said, "I feel very peaceful now because of it."

"I'm glad," he said, smiling at her, "Ariena, I'm sure you realise that spirituality is also an important aspect of the holistic paradigm, because it refers to our sense of peace."

"Yes, I do know that," she replied, "something else my mother used to say."

"I think everyone knows deep down in their hearts that spiritual awareness of our inner being will bring happiness, and with it health," he said, "but it also involves settling unresolved conflicts, forgiving and asking forgiveness, liberating toxic emotions such as anger, bitterness, hatred, resentment, regret and fear, while embracing our capacity for love, kindness, compassion and joy."

"Yes, I am already experiencing the feeling of becoming more in tune with my spiritual self, and I know I need to address these emotions to truly be free to heal completely."

"Spiritual cleansing is a process that can be achieved through various means, including meditation, affirmations, visualization and prayer," he replied, "and these strategies should be embraced as permanent lifestyle changes. You will see that the regimen becomes increasingly rewarding once healing begins and measurable results are achieved. The holistic protocol creates a physical, emotional and spiritual environment that simply will not support cancer."

"Thank you again," she said with deep feeling, as she stepped forward to give him a hug.

"You are always welcome," he replied, returning her hug, "nothing like a little infrared to finish the day! Now, off home with you, enjoy your dinner and get to bed early so you wont be falling asleep while you're here tomorrow!"

As she drove home, Ariena felt a weight of doubt and fear lift from her.

# CHAPTER 11
# RAW TRUTH

H ello, dear," Ariena's mother greeted her as she entered the kitchen, "how did your second day at the clinic go?"

"Really well, Mum," Ariena replied, kissing her on the cheek, "are you on dinner duty again?"

"It's one thing I can do to help," her mother said as she opened the oven door and pulled out a steaming casserole dish. "I've made a lovely stew with plenty of vegetables to help build your immune system," she added cheerfully.

Ariena smiled. "What's in the saucepan?" she asked, knowing not to lift the lid.

"That's the rice," her mother replied, "I've used black wild rice because it's more natural and should be better for you than white rice," she added proudly.

"It all smells delicious," Ariena said, smiling at her mother again, "and I'm really going to enjoy it, because it will be like having my last supper!"

"What do you mean, dear?" her mother turned to her with concern, "Is something wrong?"

"Oh, no Mum," Ariena replied, giving her mother a hug, "it's just that I'm going to be changing my diet as part of my healing regime, so this will be the last cooked dinner I'll be having for a while."

"Really? You mean you're going to eat everything raw?"

"Yes, exactly!"

"Well, dear," her mother took her hand and patted it, "I know that you get more nutrients from fresh raw vegetables, and fruit of course, but there are some things you have to cook to be able to eat them."

"You're absolutely right Mum," Ariena said, giving her mother's hand a squeeze, "but from what I've learnt today, it seems to me that if you have to cook food to make it digestible, then perhaps we shouldn't be eating it at all. Anyway, I need all the nutrients I can get, so I've decided, that as of tomorrow," she said, smiling as she started setting the table, "everything I eat has to be 100 per cent nutrient rich, and that means 100 per cent raw."

"Of course, we know all that, dear, but some food can be more tasty cooked than eating it raw," her mother reasoned, lifting the lid on the saucepan and stirring the rice with a fork. "Take rice for instance, you couldn't eat it uncooked."

"Exactly my point Mum," Ariena said, "so after tonight I wont be eating rice anymore."

"Okay," her mother said thoughtfully, "I guess you can get by without rice, but you need your carbohydrates, what about pasta and bread? Not to mention cakes and desserts, those are all cooked, and you do enjoy them."

"I know, but they're empty carbs Mum. Even though they might taste good, they're made of refined ingredients and then cooked at temperatures that kill any nutrients and enzymes that might have been left. It's the enzymes and nutrients that give the flavour and taste to food in it's natural state, so then we have to add sugar and spice to make it taste good!"

"Sounds crazy when you put it that way."

"It is crazy," Ariena said. "cooking food kills it, so the food is dead. Then we have to add flavouring and literally cook it to death to make it tasty. Dead food is not beneficial to the body. We need enzymes to assimilate the food, so if cooking kills the enzymes in the food, digestion will be impaired. We're living beings, so we need living food to nourish our cells if we want to live a long and healthy life, and especially if our body is already compromised," she continued, "if we continue to eat dead food, we'll all get sick and end up dead before our time. It's like meat, Mum. That's a dead animal, and you know humans shouldn't be eating animals, it's proven to be bad for our health, not to mention the health of the animals," she added ruefully.

"Hmm," her mother looked thoughtful, "yes, I do agree with you there. Studies have shown that eating red meat is very bad for your heart, and you certainly wouldn't be able to eat it raw. I'm sure that wouldn't be good for you anyway." She patted her daughter's arm again. "I remember when you were just a wee thing and you couldn't swallow meat. You chewed and chewed at it, but you couldn't swallow without gagging."

"I guess that tells you something, doesn't it?"

"Yes, well it did. I stopped giving you meat that you couldn't swallow, so long as you ate your veggies I knew you'd be healthy, so I wasn't worried."

"There you are!" Ariena exclaimed, "Anyway, I'm glad you didn't insist on my eating it, I was running out of ideas as to where to put the chewed up wad!" They both laughed.

Ariena's father put his arms out as he came through the door. "Come and give your old dad a hug," he said, kissing Ariena on the head as she snuggled into his arms. "How is my girl today?"

"Great Dad, especially now you are here."

"Glad to hear it," he said, "and I'm glad to be here. The others are just coming in too." He stepped over to Ariena's mother, putting his arm around her. "Smells like Mum's been cooking up a storm, have you love?"

"Yes, dinner is ready, get yourself cleaned up and we'll put it on the table," she said, smiling as she kissed him.

"Then will you tell us what you two were talking about?"

His wife raised her eyebrows at him, "Oh yes, have we got a surprise for you!" She looked over at her daughter and winked.

*

Ariena pushed her chair back and sighed audibly. She looked around the table at her family, her parents just finishing their meal, her son stealing the last mouthful from his sister's plate, her husband diligently mopping his plate clean with a piece of bread, and her little grandson sitting in his highchair, chewing contentedly on a piece of carrot.

"That was a big sigh love," her father said smiling at her, "hope it was a happy one?"

"Yes, Dad, it was," she answered, "I was just thinking how happy I am to be with my family right now." She looked over at her mother, "And dinner was lovely Mum, thank you."

"I'm glad you enjoyed it, dear," her mother replied with a knowing smile.

"Hey, Mum, tell us how it went at the asylum today," Scott said.

His grandmother gave him a reproachful look. "It's not an asylum, dear," she said to him, "it's a clinic."

"It's a joke, Nana," he replied laughing, "that's what they all call it there."

"Oh, I see," she said with a perplexed look.

"It's because we're all a little crazy, Mum," Ariena explained with a laugh.

"It's good to be a little crazy sometimes," her father observed, "I know I am myself!"

"And we're all crazy about you, Grandpa," Joy said, kissing his forehead as she cleared the plates from the table.

"Well, let's hear the latest news from the asylum then," he said, patting Ariena's arm.

"Okay," she said, "it was all about how I should be eating to get the best nutrition to help boost my immune system and enhance all levels of the healing process." She reached for her notebook and opened it on the table. "I made notes while the doctor was talking, so I'll go through them to make sure I cover everything," she said, "feel free to interrupt if you have any questions and hopefully I'll be able to answer them.

"As the doctor said today," she began, "it is as vital to know which foods assist in healing as it is to know which foods feed the cancer cells, so balanced body chemistry is of utmost importance for the maintenance of health and correction of dis-ease. Over-acidity in the body tissue, is one of the basic causes of most dis-ease in the body."

"Why do you say dis-ease, instead of disease?"

"I've picked that up from the good doctor," Ariena replied, "dis-ease refers to the body being in a compromised state, in other words, not being at ease. Whereas, disease refers to a specific ailment or set of symptoms that are labeled with a particular disease name, so it's identifiable for prescribed treatment or medication."

"You mentioned over-acidity, isn't that called acidosis?"

"Yes, that's a classic example," Ariena replied, "over-acidity is a symptom that tells you that the body is in a state of dis-ease. Acidosis is the name given to the symptom, which is then considered a disease, and medication can then be prescribed for it."

"Right, I get it," Glen said, "so, what you're saying is that if we treat all symptoms as disease in the body, we can take measures to find the cause and eliminate it, rather than take medication to treat the symptoms."

"Exactly, you're learning fast!" Ariena smiled at him. "You see," she continued, "a healthy body usually keeps large alkaline reserves which are used to meet the emergency demands if too many acid-producing foods are consumed, but these normal reserves can be depleted. The natural ratio in a normal healthy body is approximately 4 to 1, four parts alkaline to one part acid. When this ratio is maintained, the body has a strong resistance against dis-ease, but if the alkaline-acid ratio drops to 3 to 1, that's when your health can be in danger."

"So, does this mean that the body can only function normally and sustain health in the presence of adequate alkaline reserves, and with the proper acid-alkaline ratio in all the body tissues?"

"Yes, and the blood of course," Ariena added, "so it is vitally important that there are acid and alkaline foods in the diet. In the healing of dis-ease, the higher the ratio of alkaline elements in the diet, the faster will be the recovery. Dr Wright explained it like this; When the body digests food, it actually 'burns' the food, leaving an ash as the result of the burning, or, the digestion. This food ash can be neutral, acid or alkaline, depending largely on the mineral composition of the foods. Some foods leave an acid residue, some alkaline. The acid ash (acidosis) results when there is a depletion of the alkali reserve or the diminution in the reserve supply of fixed bases in the blood and the tissues of the body."

"Don't alkalis neutralize the acids?"

"Yes, therefore in the treatment of most dis-ease in the body, it is important that the diet includes plenty of alkaline-ash foods to offset the effects of acid-forming foods and leave a safe margin of alkalinity. So, the ideal ratio is about 80 per cent alkali-producing foods and 20 per cent acid-producing foods."

"Did Dr Wright tell you which foods are alkaline and which are acid?"

"Yes, I have a list here," Ariena replied. "There are some that are neutral ash foods and they include milk, butter, cheese, vegetable oils and white sugar. Neutral ash foods eventually have the same effect in the body of creating dis-ease, but are generally non-symptomatic at the time of eating them. In other words, they don't usually cause acidosis, but over time, the affect from eating these foods will accumulate and create dis-ease in the body."

"So many people have allergies to dairy products these days," Joy commented, "but it's not really an allergy is it?"

"The fact is," Ariena replied, "we're just not meant to eat dairy products, our bodies aren't designed to assimilate it as food. Cow's milk is for baby cows, just like human mother's milk is for human babies, it's the perfect food in both cases. Calves grow at a rapid rate compared to human babies, so their mother's milk is perfect for them," she explained, "and as we can see with our little Kenny here, his mother's milk is perfect for him."

"Yes," her daughter agreed, "I'm really glad to be still nursing him, we all know that it gives a child the best start in life to have his own mother's milk."

"I never figured out why so many people think they still need to drink milk as adults," Glen chipped in, "in their natural environment, no other adult animals drink their mother's milk after they have weaned themselves."

"For that matter," Scott joined in, "only humans drink milk from another animal species anyway, what's with that?"

"That's because animals are smarter than us," his father replied. "Animals that are still living in their natural environment are still living intuitively, they don't need to go to university to learn how to live, they already know. It's when we put them in an unnatural environment and feed them the wrong food, that they get sick, like us."

"You're right son," his father-in-law said, "ever since farmers changed from the old way of farming to the terrible agribusiness of feedlots and factory farming, the poor animals have become sick, and so have we."

"We even put our pets at risk," his wife added, "you don't see lions and tigers, or wolves taking themselves off to the vet, like we have to with our pet cats and dogs when we give them canned food."

"Yes, you're all right," Ariena agreed, "we have been brainwashed by the meat and dairy board, and other animal industries, to believe that it's healthy for us, but there is so much evidence from medical studies now that shows in fact it's the reverse. All animal products are bad for our health, and of course, extremely bad for the animal's health. There's a lot more to agribusiness and factory farming than you would care to know, there's the whole cruelty issue, and of course, that extends to the pharmaceutical and chemical industries as well as the cosmetic industries. Experimentation on animals in the name of research for human health and ego is unnecessary and therefore completely inexcusable. So, apart from it being unhealthy for humans to eat other animals, or use animal products in any form, it has become a compassionate issue as well."

Despite taking a deep breath to try to control her emotions, a tear escaped and rolled down Ariena's cheek. Her mother quickly stood up and came around the table to give her a hug.

"The more I think about it, the more I feel ashamed to be human," she said, wiping her daughter's cheek with her handkerchief.

"Thanks, Mum," Ariena said, smiling at her, "I'm sorry, I'm a bit emotional these days."

"I can understand that, dear," she replied, wiping away a tear from her own cheek, "it's hard, but we do have to think of these things to be able to make change in this world."

"I'll put the kettle on," Ariena's father said, getting up from the table, "a nice pot of chamomile tea will do us all good."

"Thanks, Grandpa, that's just what we need. Let's go into the living room and sit in the comfy chairs while you tell us the rest," Scott suggested, lifting his nephew out of the highchair, "come on Kenny, you can play on the floor while we talk."

*

Ariena settled herself into the chair nearest a small table where she placed her notes. "Okay, we were up to acid forming foods," she said, referring to the notes and continuing, "so we know these include all red meat, including veal, liver and all organ meats, as well as chicken, fowl and eggs, oysters and most fish. Lentils, peanuts, and most nuts except almonds and Brazil are also acid forming. Other acid forming foods are rice, bread, even wholewheat or rye, and obviously wheat and white flour. In fact," she continued, "most grains are acid-forming except millet and buckwheat, which are considered to be alkaline because they are actually seeds."

"Doesn't sprouting grains make them more alkaline?"

"Yes, soaking nuts, seeds and grains releases the enzyme inhibitors that are acid forming to us, and the sprouting process is the life force that is alkaline, as it is then a living food."

"So, we should be soaking all our nuts and seeds before we eat them, even if we want to eat them raw?"

"Yes, you soak them and rinse them until the rinse water is clear, then you know the enzyme inhibitors are released."

"What are the enzyme inhibitors for?"

"That is nature's way of safe guarding the seed until it is in the perfect environment to sprout and start living as a new plant."

"Good old Mother Nature has everything figured out."

"Sure has," Ariena agreed, smiling at her father's comment, "if we follow Mother Nature's teachings, everything would be in balance and we'd all be well. We just have to get back to the natural way of things."

"Yes," her mother agreed, "that's the way nature intended it to be. If everyone were to think more consciously about the choices they make in life, the world would be a healthier place." She stood up and walked back into the kitchen.

"Mum, are you okay?" Ariena called.

"Yes, dear," her mother replied as she returned with bowl of fresh fruit and put it on the table. "Help yourselves to some alkaline dessert," she said, handing an apple to her great-grandson. "Here you go little man," she said. Kenny's eyes lit up as he reached out and took the apple from her, biting into it immediately and munching loudly with a big grin on his face.

"Kids know intuitively what food is good for them," Joy commented, "until we feed them other foods and they lose their intuitive abilities. I mean, they even chew on grass like the animals do, until we tell them not to."

"Good point, sis," Scott said, "I remember we used to make mud pies, decorate them with grass and flowers, and then eat them! They didn't taste that good, but I don't think we got sick from it, did we Mum?"

Ariena laughed. "No, you didn't get sick from eating your little creations," she recalled with a smile, "but I remember you changed to pretending to eat them after you tried them a few times."

"It was the dirt," Joy said, "too gritty. Still, I guess we got a few minerals from it."

"Yeah, and vitamin B12," Scott added, "you don't worry about Kenny eating dirt, do you?"

"No, of course not," she replied, "it's self regulating. He only eats it until he finds something better, like grass, or Mum's flowers in the garden!"

"Animals that virtually live on grass are getting all the nutrients they need from the greens and grass they eat," her grandmother commented, "so I don't think eating grass will do him any harm, dear."

"Wait till you hear what I found out today about grass!" Ariena said.

"We're not going to start eating grass are we?" Scott asked.

"No, not eating it," she replied, "our bodies can't assimilate grass because it has so much cellulose in it, we'd need another stomach or two like the cows have, but we can juice it and drink it."

"That's why ruminants chew their cud all day, to break down the cellulose."

"Really Nana? I thought they were meditating."

"That too, my dear," his grandmother replied, "we can learn a lot from animals. Animals know instinctively what and how to eat to stay healthy. They don't need to go to school or university to learn how to live, and they don't need doctors and hospitals because they take care of themselves. Animals don't cook their food and they don't have all the health problems we do. When you think about it, they eat all their food live and raw, even the carnivores," she added, "which doesn't bear thinking about, really."

"No, it doesn't," Ariena agreed, "but they are designed to eat that way, we're not. Otherwise we'd have teeth and stomachs and intestines of a carnivore, but we don't. Our bodies are designed to eat living plant food, like the other herbivores."

"That's a good point. When you think of all the plant eating animals, they are certainly very healthy," her mother said.

"Yep, all the largest, tallest and strongest land animals live on plants, and they don't have any health problems, not even with their bones and muscles, so therefore they are getting all the nutrients that they need, including calcium and protein," Ariena said, "and, don't forget, the elephant is also said to have the best memory!"

Her mother smiled. "Exactly, but what about the most energetic animal! They don't call it the energiser bunny for nothing! Just think of the rate at which they multiply, those little guys could well be the most intelligent as well!" They all laughed.

"Tell us about the alkaline foods, dear," Ariena's father said.

"Well, all fresh fruits and vegetables are alkaline ash foods, but some are more so than others. The most alkaline fruits are figs, apricots, dates, and raisins, cantaloupe, pineapple, grapefruit, peaches, tomatoes, cucumber, apples, grapes, bananas and watermelon. The most alkaline veggies are spinach and all leafy greens, turnip and beet tops, carrots, celery and lettuce, watercress and potatoes," she took a breath and continued, "almonds, Brazil nuts, coconuts, millet, and buckwheat, together with fresh vegetable and fruit juices are also highly alkaline."

"That's why Nana eats almonds and Brazil nuts every day."

"I read in one of my health books that they help prevent cancer, I'm sure they would help get rid of it too," her mother said smiling at Ariena.

"Yep, well, I'll be including them in my regime from now on," Ariena said.

"So, what about the juices, what are the most alkali-forming?"

Ariena looked back at her list, "All green grasses, juices of beets and tops, carrot, celery, fig, pineapple and citrus juices," she replied.

"Sounds like the makings of a good soup," her father said.

"Well, vegetable broth is also an extremely alkalizing drink," she replied, "but when you cook the vegetables, most of the nutrients will be lost, so juicing the vegetables is a better option."

"I see," her father pondered for a moment then added, "so it's soup in a glass."

"That's right Grandpa, you can drink your soup instead of slurping it off your spoon!" said Scott.

"Ahh, but that's the best part young man," his grandfather replied.

"You could always use a straw to drink the soup juice, has the same sound effects!"

"Good idea!" he replied with a wink and a nod. They all laughed at the thought of it.

\*

"I noticed you included tomatoes and cucumber with the fruit."

"Yes, well technically, they are a fruit. We tend to think of them as vegetables because we eat them with other vegetables, but if it has a seed, it's a fruit."

"That's interesting, I never thought of it that way."

"So, you were serious about drinking grass juice?"

"Absolutely," Ariena replied, "the immune system works better when the body is fully hydrated, so drinking pure water and herbal teas, raw fruit and vegetable juices, especially grass juices, together with an abundance of organic plant foods rich in nutrients, is essential to provide layers of nutritional protection."

"Great! If we juice the grass every day, I wont have to mow the lawns," Glen said enthusiastically.

Ariena smiled. "I think we'll have to grow the grass specially for juicing," she said, "but I've got some information on that as well, so I'll get to that in a minute. Meanwhile, let's get back to the food that we put in our system, since that determines the health of every cell and organ in the body." Ariena took a banana out of the bowl and started peeling it. She broke off the top and handed it to her mother, who offered it to her great grandson.

"Ta, nana, Nana," he said, laughing at his little joke. Ariena took a bite and passed the remaining banana to her daughter. "Give him the rest when he's finished that piece love," she said, picking up her notes.

The little boy clapped his hands and chuckled again as he said, "More nana, Mama!"

"As I mentioned before," Ariena said, "with cancer, it's particularly important to know what foods help boost the immune system and which foods feed the cancer. So I'll be eliminating all foods that have a negative affect and increasing the foods that have a positive affect on my health."

"Before you go on, dear," her mother interrupted, putting her hand on Ariena's arm, "I want to say something."

"Sure Mum, go ahead."

"Well, I've been doing some research of my own about maintaining health through nutrition," she announced, "and from what I've read, it is just as crucial to eat the right food to prevent dis-ease in the body, as it is to eat the right food for healing cancer, or any other health issue for that matter. So, I wanted to say, that whatever changes you make in your diet, I'll be making them too, *and*, I think we all should."

"Aww, Mum," Ariena took her mother's hand and squeezed it, "you don't have to…"

"Yes, I do," her mother contradicted her. "I want to support you in every way I can, and this is a very easy thing to do. After all, if you can do it, so can I," she looked around her family and added, "we all can."

"It may not be as easy as you think, Mum," Ariena said.

"How hard can it be? If it's just eliminating everything that's negative and increasing everything that is positive, it's not compli-cated. Anyway, if I'm going to be helping with the meals while you are having therapy, I might as well be making them all the same for everyone, *and* it will be good for all of us to make these changes," her mother replied.

"I'm happy with any meals you make, love," Ariena's father said, patting his wife's arm.

"Me too, Mum," Glen said. "I agree, in supporting Ariena, we can all be improving our own health at the same time. You're not alone in this," he added turning to Ariena and kissing her cheek, "this is a wake-up call for all of us. We all need to take responsibil-ity for our own health, *and* for our children's." He bent down and kissed his grandson on his head.

"Us too, right sis?' Scott chimed in.

"Yep, we're all in this together Mum," Joy replied, standing up and giving Ariena a hug.

"That's what a family is all about," Ariena's father commented, "pass me the fruit bowl!" He took a banana and started peeling it.

Kenny looked up and clapped his hands, "More nana, Grampa."

"Well, that's unanimous then," he laughed.

Ariena wiped a tear from her eye. "I love you all so much," she said tearfully.

Her grandson looked up at her and asked, "Nannie sad?"

"No, darling, Nannie is very happy," Ariena told him.

"Story, Nannie," he said, climbing on her lap and reaching over to take the banana from her father's hand.

"You know what you want, don't you wee fella," he said, and turning to his daughter he said, "Come on sweetheart, tell us a story."

\*

"Okay," Ariena said, "here's what has been recommended. First, refined salt and sugar feeds and strengthens cancer cells so should be eliminated. Everything that can weaken the immune system must also be avoided, so that means all sugary starchy foods, sugar substitutes and refined flour. Also, all hydrogenated oils, saturated fats and trans fatty acids, all processed foods, including carbonated drinks, coffee and alcohol, as they all damage the body and numerous studies link them to cancer. Obviously, as we've already discussed," she added, "meats and animal products, including dairy and all mucus-forming foods should also be avoided." She stopped to look at everyone, and noted the look of interest on everyone's face as they listened intently. "Elements such as chlorine and fluoride also interfere with healing and may fuel cancer growth," she continued, "so we need to be filtering the water or getting fresh spring water."

"I've heard of a place up on the mountain road where people take their bottles and collect the fresh spring water, maybe we should look into it," Scott suggested.

"Sounds like a good job for you, batman." his father said.

"I have a question," Ariena's father said, "if we are to eliminate meat and all animal products entirely, where do we get our protein?"

"That's a good question Dad," she replied, "let me tell you a story about the protein myth."

*

"Next to water, protein is the most plentiful nutrient in the body. More than 50 per cent of the dry weight of the body is protein," she began. "Proteins are composed of smaller protein chains called amino acids, and amino acids are the raw building materials of the body whilst enzymes do the actual building. So together, enzymes and amino acids are responsible for cell renewal and a huge array of diverse functions from the creation of hormones to building of muscles, blood and organs."

"Isn't it the amino acids that are responsible for the rapid healing of cuts and wounds?"

"Yes, and for proper liver function, and digestion and assimilation of foods."

"I've read that amino acids also regulate mental awareness levels," Ariena's mother added.

"That's why I'm concerned about getting enough protein, dear," her husband replied, "what with my memory loss and all."

"Well Dad," Ariena said, "proteins are able to unite with either acid or alkaline substances to aid the body in maintaining proper acid-alkaline balance of the blood and the tissues for strong immunity against all dis-ease in the body. Of the 22 different kinds of amino acids," she continued, "there are eight that the body does not manufacture, and nine in babies," she added kissing her grandson on the nose, "and they can only be synthesized from the proteins we eat. They are called the essential amino acids. If these amino acids are not present in the diet, the body is unable to rejuvenate cells properly and deficiency symptoms arise."

"Okay, go on."

"Now, as we know, it has been widely taught that animal products such as meat, dairy and eggs are the best source of protein, as they contain large amounts of all eight essential amino acids and are therefore called complete protein. Whereas," she continued, "individual plant foods are called incomplete proteins because they do not contain all eight essential amino acids. There is of course, the exception of soybeans and wheatgrass, which are also complete proteins," she added, "however, the eight essential and at least fourteen nonessential amino acids *are* found in various plants in generous amounts."

"Ahh, so there lies the myth," her father said with a nod of comprehension, "that without meat and dairy the body cannot build muscle nor retain energy."

"Yes, exactly," Scott said joining in, "it is a myth which has been based on the incorrect interpretation of complete and incomplete protein."

"Right," his sister agreed. "Complete protein does not mean the most important, or that it's better than an incomplete protein."

"Sounds like it's become far more complicated than it really is."

"Exactly! Foods containing all eight essential amino acids are called complete protein, and foods that do *not* contain all the essential amino acids are called incomplete protein. It's that simple!"

"So, we've been lead to believe all these years that meat and dairy and eggs are essential for our health because they are complete proteins, and that plant based food is inferior for our health because it is an incomplete protein."

"Yep, that's right."

"If you ask me, that's wrong! I mean, how could they make such a mistake?"

"I don't think it was a mistake, Grandpa, meat, dairy and egg production are big industries."

"Now that there are so many studies showing meat and dairy are causing all kinds of disease, I mean *dis-ease* in the body, it's also been to the detriment of our health!" He turned to his daughter, "You better tell us more about getting our protein from plants, dear."

\*

"Well, when you eat a variety of plant foods throughout the day, the various amounts of amino acids in the foods combine to make the eight essential amino acids," Ariena said. "Proteins are abundant in foods derived from plants, and they have the added benefit of being naturally cholesterol free, high in fibre and low in fat."

"That sounds good, but what if you get too little protein?"

"Protein deficiency is almost unknown worldwide in humans, Dad," she replied, "but protein excess is a real problem in developed societies. For instance, in North America and Australia most people eat too much protein, they eat an average of 160 grams of protein daily, which is about 8 times what they need. So, you see, when you eat a diet that includes meat, dairy and eggs, it is easy to get too much protein, which is another good reason to get your protein from plant foods."

"What is the ideal intake of protein for a human being?"

"'Ideally, 20-40 grams per day," Ariena replied, "but the average North American and Australian adult consumes 90 to 120 grams of protein per day, and that is without going on a high protein diet! This is because they consume large amounts of meat, dairy products and eggs, which are already very high in protein."

"I read the other day that according to the World Health Organisation, the maximum total daily protein intake the body needs is 8 per cent of the total daily calories," Joy added, "so if people are getting enough calories, they are virtually certain to be getting enough protein." Her little son, hearing Joy's voice, squirmed off Ariena's lap and toddled over to her.

"Boobie, Mama," he said, as he climbed onto her lap.

"Out of the mouths of babes," Ariena said with a laugh, "I was just going to say that the greatest point to be made about the protein issue, comes from Mother Nature herself. You see, human mother's milk provides 5 per cent of its calories as protein. So, nature seems to be telling us that little babies, whose bodies are growing the fastest they will ever grow in their lives and whose protein needs are maximum, are best served when 5 per cent of their food calories come as protein."

"Every expert in the field of nutrition has talked about the protein requirements for babies and their growth, versus adults' needs," Joy said, stroking her son's hair as he suckled, "and at no other time will the body be developing and growing as fast as during babyhood. That's when bone growth, brain growth, teeth, nails, hair and every cell and muscle in the body are growing at the speed of light."

"Exactly," agreed her brother, "even bodybuilders do not grow muscle as fast as a newborn baby. Do you know that most of the well-known bodybuilders say that the protein requirements of a bodybuilder is only 1 gram of protein for every 2 pounds of body weight, and that can come from basic good eating, People tend to go overboard on protein, something I believe to be totally unnecessary."

"Too true," Ariena agreed, "and to meet those protein requirements, one can do fine without meat, dairy products and eggs. I mean, eating only broccoli, you'd get three times the quota suggested!"

"Good, I love broccoli," Scott replied, "what other plant foods have protein?"

"All unrefined plant foods are loaded with proteins," Ariena replied, "the most common sources of plant protein are wheatgrass juice, dark leafy greens, soybeans, nuts, pumpkin, rice, beans and lentils, sunflower and sesame seeds, corn, potatoes, oranges and dates, the list goes on and on."

"From what I was reading," Ariena's mother joined in, "animal foods are dangerously high in protein, which contributes to kidney damage leading to kidney stones, and protein metabolism especially taxes the kidneys and liver."

"That's right, Mum," Ariena agreed, "when protein content of the diet exceeds 15 per cent of calories consumed, the body's liver and kidneys are burdened with the task of removing the excess amounts of protein. A high protein diet imposes a workload on the entire digestive system," she continued, "which may contribute to feelings of fatigue and lack of energy. There's also been recent studies to show that a high protein diet can irritate the immune system, and aggravate dis-ease such as rheumatoid arthritis and lupus, causing the immune system to mistakenly attack the body's own tissues."

"Well, we all know that eating animal foods can cause heart problems because of the high amounts of cholesterol and saturated fat," her mother added, "so a high protein diet creates a higher risk for developing heart disease, hypertension, diabetes and cancer. It's also been proven that the diuretic effect of high protein intake leaches minerals out of the body, resulting in phosphorus and calcium deficiency. Loss of calcium from bones can produce the condition known as osteoporosis."

"Yes," Ariena agreed, "and we're told to increase the intake of calcium by drinking cow's milk, whereas osteoporosis is less a condition of calcium deficiency, than one of protein excess. The studies show that osteoporosis tends to occur in countries where calcium intake through dairy products is highest. We are better to get calcium from plant source such as dark greens, sea vegetables, figs, nuts, sesame and flax seeds."

"Seems like we've been led up the wrong path by the dairy board again," her father said, "so if meat and dairy products, and eggs you say, are now proven to be unhealthy foods, why do they keep telling us we need them, don't they know?"

"Of course they know, Grandpa. It's not just the dairy board, the whole animal industry has been lying to us for years. Think about it for a minute, if everyone stopped eating meat, dairy and eggs, there wouldn't be an animal industry."

"But, what about people's health?"

"They're not concerned about people's health Gramps, it's all about making money."

"Do you think," the old man pondered, "do you think that they're in cohoots with the pharmaceutical industry?"

"Now you're starting to realise what's going on, dear," his wife said, "of course they are. Truth be known, they're probably run by them. If we keep eating foods that are unhealthy, eventually they make us sick, so we go to the doctor and he gives us a prescription, and the pharmaceutical industry sells more medication. They're in cohoots all right, mark my words!" Ariena raised her eyebrows and smiled at the others.

"I've just thought of something else," her father said, "do you think the doctors are in on this?"

"I'm sure they are being paid by the pharmaceutical industry to push their drugs Gramps, they're probably on a commission."

"Wow, I've just thought of something else," his grandfather said, "maybe we're being given medication that we don't really need."

"I keep telling you that you don't need all those pills," his wife said, and turning to the others she shook her head, "every week when we go to town, he goes to see the doctor while I'm having my hair done, and that old codger gives him all kinds of pills."

"Why do you go to see the doctor every week, Dad? You're not ill are you?"

"No, love," her father replied, "he's an old friend, I just go for a chat while I'm waiting for your Mum."

"And he gives you pills to take? What are they for?"

"I was having trouble sleeping because my old legs get cramp when I lie down, so he gave me some for that, and some for my memory loss, but I don't know what the others are for, he gives me different ones each week, says I should try them."

"Oh, you're kidding," Ariena shook her head, "how many are we talking about?"

"There are lots, but I don't let him take them all," her mother said, "I told him it's too many."

"I think we better have a look, Dad," Ariena said, still shaking her head, "I'll come over tomorrow and we can go through them and identify what they are for."

"Okay, love, that's a good idea."

"I've told him, it's not right," her mother continued, "I think they're using the old folks to experiment on, I won't have any of it. I do make sure we have our multi-vitamins though." Everyone smiled.

"Good on you, Nana," Joy said, "but maybe once you're getting more nutrients from the food you eat, you wont need to take them either. Some of those vitamin pills have all sorts of fillers and things added to them that aren't good for you either."

"You could be right there, dear," she replied."

"Yeah, the old way of farming where the cows are free to roam in fields of fresh, green grass is fast disappearing," Scott joined in, "in the feed lots the animals are fed inappropriate and altered food that is laced with all kinds of chemicals, and, not only that, they're feeding them pellets made from the animals that have died from being sick! That's what caused mad cow's disease, feeding animals contaminated meat," he added with disgust.

"Sounds more like mad human's disease to me," his grandfather commented.

"You're right there, Dad," Glen said, coming into the discussion, "but even if the cows do graze in fields, the pesticides and airborne pollution settles on the grass, and it's ingested and becomes imbedded into the tissues. Then when humans eat these animal products, the pollutants and poisons are also consequently ingested, another reason to get protein from plant foods I'd say!" Ariena looked at her husband and smiled.

"Well, if all these reasons are not enough, there is always the simple reason of cost," she said, "it's much more cost efficient to eat just fresh fruit and vegetables, and some protein rich nuts and seeds, especially if we grow most of them ourselves or buy them direct from the organic farmers, than to buy meats, eggs and dairy products as well. Of course," she continued, "if you compare the cost to our health of a diet laden with saturated fat, cholesterol and excessive protein, to a healthy nutrient rich diet, there is no comparison."

"What about comparing the cost to the *planet* of the environmental consequences of human food choices," Joy commented. "The Food & Agriculture Organisation of the United Nations recently released a report called 'Livestock's Long Shadow' which states that animal industries are one of the 'most significant contributors to the most serious environmental problems, at every scale from local to global'. Animal industries have a negative impact on bio-diversity through pollution and habitat destruction, and the introduction of non-native species with increased competition for food and water."

"How does it affect water consumption, dear?" her grandfather asked.

"Well, Grandpa," she replied, "raising animals for food requires enormous amounts of water, it takes 50,000 litres of water to produce 1 kilogram of beef!

"Wow, that's incredible!"

"Yes, but it only takes 2,500 litres to produce 1 kilogram of grain and much less for fruits and vegetables," she continued, "so reducing meat and dairy consumption is the most effective way to reduce water use."

"Did you know that over 30 per cent of greenhouse emissions produced can be attributed to animal industries," her brother said, "there's a recent University study that compared the indirect energy use associated with animal and plant-based diets. It found that adopting a plant-based diet would save substantially greater carbon dioxide emissions than switching from a regular car to a hybrid car. So, it would not only make a real difference to our health, but also the health of the planet."

*

"Okay, I'm sold," their grandfather said, "tell me what veggies we need and I'll start growing them in the garden, and your Nana can cook them up for dinner."

"Um, Gramps, you didn't hear the part about what happens to food when you cook it?"

"*I'll* be growing it young fella, it's your Nana who will be cooking it."

"Preparing it, dear," his wife corrected him, "I'll be preparing it. I think it's time for you to explain," she said to Ariena.

"Yes, I guess so," she agreed, "you see Dad, the human body needs live foods to build live cells. Fruits and vegetables fresh from the garden come directly from the soil and for this reason, they are considered to be live foods. There is a vast quantity of evidence showing that a high raw diet, a way of eating in which 80 per cent of your foods are eaten raw, or uncooked, not only reverses the bodily degeneration which accompanies long term illness, but makes you feel better emotionally, increases your energy levels and even retards the rate at which you age!"

"Sounds good so far," her father commented, "especially if it slows down aging. Are there any particular foods that you should be eating for the cancer though, love?"

"All plant foods contain nutrients that aid healing," she replied, "but herbs, fruits and vegetables have properties that inhibit the proliferation of cancer, and protect against it, while at the same time, cleanse, repair and strengthen the body. Plant foods that are known to be particularly helpful when cancer is present include all the cruciferous vegetables like broccoli, cauliflower and cabbage, all green leafy vegetables, all fruits, but especially berries and dark grapes with seeds and skins, garlic, ginger, and turmeric."

"Isn't it hard to digest cruciferous vegetables? I've heard it's best to cook broccoli for instance."

"At first it may be best to lightly blanch or steam them, until you are used to eating them raw," Ariena replied, "but it is important to chew raw food well, which has the same effect of breaking it down that steaming has. Also, whole foods such as avocados, nuts and seeds provide the essential fatty acids necessary for oxygenation of cells, but they should be kept to a minimum, approximately 10 per cent of the diet, since fat slows digestion and in large quantities may accelerate tumor growth. So, aiming for a diet that is at least 80 per cent raw, will ensure an alkaline environment as well as an ample supply of enzymes for the healing process."

"So do you still have three meals a day, or is there a different protocol for eating this diet?"

"Well, making the change to eating mostly raw fruits and vegetables may make you feel hungry, because you body is used to having bulk three times a day, " Ariena explained, "so you should eat small meals three, four or even five times during the day. You start the day with a nourishing green smoothie, or fresh fruit, but consume most of your daily food intake in the morning and afternoon, and eat very little in the evening. If you are hungry in the evening before bed, eat fresh fruit, as it is easy and quick to digest."

"One of the biggest mistakes most people make is to eat heavy food late in the day," her mother added, "your body doesn't want to be digesting food as you sleep."

"No, your entire system should have uninterrupted, restful time to rejuvenate, detoxify, purify and regenerate."

"Okay, so no more cornflakes for breakfast I take it. I'm not sure about your green smoothies though." "It's just fruit and greens blended up, you'll love it Gramps."

"If you say so, and we have the main meal of the day at lunch time?"

"Yep, exactly. You can have one of Nana's beautiful mixed salads, all fresh from your garden."

"No more sliced boiled eggs on top though," her mother smiled.

"There are also some great recipes for raw dishes you can try," Ariena said, "like raw veggie lasagne, you can adapt all your favourite dishes quite easily."

"This sounds exciting," her mother said, "I'll have to get more recipe books!"

"So, what do you snack on between meals? No more crisps out of a packet I guess."

"Right Dad," Ariena smiled at her father, "but you can have a few pieces of dried fruit or soaked nuts, or sprouted seeds and of course, fresh fruit. Then, for dinner, you can have a small portion of raw salad with a glass of carrot or other vegetable juice, or you can have a light fruit smoothie or a selection of fresh fruit, or eat just one fruit like a papaya or melon."

"You mean I can eat a whole melon all to myself?"

"Sure, why not?"

"I'm liking this idea already!" her father laughed, "but what about if we go out to eat, like at a restaurant."

"You do what I've been doing for years as a vegetarian," she replied, "order a salad, but ask for extra veggies including avocado, and ask for lemon wedges instead of salad dressing," she added, "dressings are usually processed or may have egg and dairy products in them. If you squeeze the lemon on the salad yourself, then you know it's fresh, and the avocado gives a creamy consistency to the salad."

"Restaurants don't always have avocado on the menu though."

"You can always take an avocado along to add to the salad in case the restaurant does not have it available, I always have one in my bag."

"What about when it's cold, like in winter," he asked, "aren't we going to want hot food to warm us up?"

"Well, actually Dad, that's a bit of a fallacy," Ariena replied, smiling at her father. "I mean, when there's a frost on the ground in the morning, we don't go outside to eat breakfast, and when it's snowing out we don't eat lunch or dinner on the deck. We're inside where it's warm."

"True," he agreed, nodding slightly, "but if you've been outside in the cold and you come in, it's very comforting to have a hot bowl of soup, or one of Nana's delicious curry stews to warm you up."

"Is that where the expression 'comfort food' comes from?"

"Yes, it's the idea that certain foods make you feel warm and comfortable."

"In reality Grandpa, you can't eat really hot food anyway. That's why you blow on it to cool it down so you can put it in your mouth, otherwise it would burn you."

"Or slurp it noisily if it's soup!" They all laughed.

"You're right though, I've never really thought about it, you can't eat or drink hot food, but it is nice to put your cold hands around a warm cup of soup, *and* slurp it!" he added, winking at his granddaughter.

"There's no reason why you couldn't warm up a raw vegetable soup Dad, so long as you don't cook all the goodness out of it,"

Ariena said. "If you want to warm the food, just keep the temperature below 37 degrees, then the nutrients and enzymes are still intact. It's when we boil or cook food in a hot oven that the value of the food is compromised."

"Could I use the microwave?"

"No Gramps! That nukes it! You definitely need to throw your microwave away!"

"Oh, dear, no cooking and no microwave? What will we put in it's place?"

"Nana's new recipe books of course! Don't worry Gramps, we'll take care of the microwave while you take Nana shopping."

"This may seem like a lot at first, Dad," Ariena said, putting her arm around her father's shoulder, "and it may take a while to build up to eating 80 per cent raw food, but you'll soon find that you will begin to feel more healthy, so it will get easier."

"Yeah Grandpa, soon you'll be so full of energy, we wont be able to keep up with you!"

"I'm sure you are right," he replied, giving his daughter a kiss, "it's just a bit overwhelming, but I'm willing to try anything if it will help improve your health, and sounds like it will improve my health too. So whatever it takes, it's better than doing nothing."

"Good on you, Grandpa, guess you can teach an old dog new tricks, hey?"

"You're never to old to learn, young man, I'll be the first to say that, and it's never too late to make changes for the better either."

\*

Ariena's daughter stood up, her little son sleeping soundly in her arms. "I'm going to pop him on your bed so we can stay and hear about fasting and juicing," Joy said as she left the room.

"Yes, the idea of juicing sounds great," Scott said, "especially juicing grass, eh Dad?"

"Yep, might as well try everything son," his father agreed, "and like I said, I'd rather be juicing it than mowing it!" Joy returned to the room and settled herself on the couch next to her father.

"Knowing you Dad, you'll be growing and selling it next," she laughed.

"Now, that's not a bad idea, sweetheart," he replied thoughtfully. She raised her eyebrows at her brother and winked.

"Okay Mum," she said, turning to her mother. "What's the deal with fasting and juicing?"

Ariena smiled. "Well apparently," Ariena began, "an effective way to boost the immune system is to cleanse the body internally through fasting, or not eating at all."

"I hope you're not suggesting we stop eating altogether, are you?" her father said to her with a look of apprehension.

"No Dad," she replied, giving him a reassuring smile, "fasting can be highly beneficial for reversing dis-ease in the body, it allows the body to rest from digesting food and therefore gives it a chance to rejuvenate. but it can also be beneficial to fast before and during the transition to eating a raw food diet."

"We're actually fasting while we sleep, that's where the name for the first meal of the day comes from," her mother said.

"Anyway, I'm going to start out by not eating one day per week, only drinking water and fresh raw juices throughout that day," Ariena continued, "and if I feel the need for something to eat during my fast day, I'll have some grapes, they help to move things out."

"I've heard that some people just fast on water only, and for a long period of time," her mother said, "you're not going to do that are you?"

"No Mum," Ariena assured her, "I need to keep nourishing the body right now, so a water fast would not be a good idea. However, a juice fast would be very beneficial."

"You mean just drinking juice?"

"If I was going to fast for any length of time, yes," she replied, "but meanwhile, I'll be including several juices a day in my regime, based on a couple of therapies that I've discussed with my doctor."

"Is that the Gerson Therapy and the Breuss Cancer Cure?" Glen asked. "I saw you have been reading those books."

"Yes, that's right," she replied, "both therapies were established years ago and have been highly successful in reversing cancer, so there's nothing to lose by including them as well as the immune therapy."

"Nothing to lose, except cancer," her mother stated, "and everything to gain."

"Exactly Mum," Ariena agreed, "The benefits of detoxification or internal cleansing are numerous, it allows the body to rid itself of toxins that have accumulated in many forms, like preservatives, colourings and other additives to our foods, and heavy metals and chemicals that we've been exposed to at work or home, not to mention the residue from any prescription drugs that you've had over the years. Anyway, freshly squeezed juices make up a vital part of any detox or cleansing program. They have a powerful effect, stimulating the whole system and encouraging the elimination of toxins, and that's what I need to do."

"I'm sure we can all do with some detoxing," her mother said, "and drinking juice is an easy way to do it. We'll have to get a good juicer along with the raw recipe books!"

"This shopping spree is starting to worry my wallet," Ariena's father said, "can't we just buy the juice with the other groceries?"

"No Dad," Ariena replied, "fresh raw juice is different from bottled, canned or concentrated juices sold in the supermarket.

First, it is absolutely fresh, which is important because nutrients lose value soon after juicing, and second, fresh juice is not pasteurized like the store bought juices, which is a process that kills living cells that are so vital to good health. Raw juice is absolutely pure, free of the additives and preservatives, which are highly toxic to the body that are also in store bought juices."

"Okay, so you're saying we have to get a juicer and juice the vegetables ourselves."

"That's right."

"Why can't we just eat more vegetables, wont that do the job?"

"No one can physically eat enough raw foods to nourish their body correctly," Ariena replied, "we would have to consume about seven kilograms of raw organic plants every day to supply the body with what it needs, but one cup of raw carrot juice contains the equivalent nutrient value of four cups of raw chopped carrots, and you would never sit down and eat that many carrots at once," she explained. "Not only that, you can drink several cups of juice a day, so, by doing so, your nutrition level increases exponentially. Also, when made fresh and consumed immediately, juices contain about 95 per cent of the food value of fruits and vegetables and instantly release nourishment to the body through the bloodstream. In the process," she continued, "the body receives all the necessary nutrients, vitamins and minerals. When we eat fresh fruit and vegetables, the chewing process acts just like a juicer. Our bodies extract the liquid which contains all the nutrients that we need, from the fibre, and that passes into the lower digestive tract to be eliminated. The extracted liquid has the same elements as fresh raw juice that you make in a juicer."

"So, by drinking raw juice, you are eliminating a digestive process and efficiently supplying the body with a purely healthful and natural way to get all its nutritional needs," Scott joined in.

"Yes, nutrient rich juice supplies our cells with everything they need to stay healthy and functioning. According to the books on juicing therapies I've been reading," his mother continued, "it cleanses our systems and strengthens bones, contributes to a healthy heart and makes your hair shine!"

"Having shiny hair is certainly preferable to loosing all your hair, like you would have if you'd had chemotherapy," Joy commented.

"Okay, that all makes sense, we'll get a juicer so you can have the juice fresh."

\*

"There's one other thing you mentioned earlier that we need to know more about," Joy said, "better tell us about the wheatgrass juice."

"Wait till you hear this Grandpa," Scott said, giving his grandfather a gentle push.

"Listen, young fella, if I can juice it, we can drink it," he replied, tussling his grandson's hair. "Tell us all about it, love," he said, patting Ariena's arm, "what with all these carrots and greens, if we're going to be eating rabbit food, we might as well include the grass!"

"Okay, I'll be brief because it's getting late," Ariena said, "and we all need our sleep. So, as we mentioned before, wheatgrass is known as a complete protein because it contains the eight essential amino acids, as well as seventeen other amino acids. Along with the essential amino acids, wheatgrass juice also contains alamine – a blood builder, asparic acid, which improves mental balance and serine which stimulates brain and nerve function. When grown in organic soil wheatgrass absorbs 92 per cent of the known 102 minerals from the soil and contains all the vitamins that science has isolated. Wheatgrass also contains live enzymes, and is, therefore, a complete food."

"You mentioned enzymes before, but what are they required for?"

"Wheatgrass juice is high in active enzymes which are needed for everything we do." Ariena replied. "All our vital functions, such as breathing, digestion, vision and reproduction, even our thoughts and dreams, are all controlled by enzymes. Each enzyme performs a specific function within the body while in harmony with other enzymes," she added, "they have also been linked to the prevention and curing of cancer. When I was at the asylum today," she smiled at her own use of the word, "I was reading an article published in the Journal of Longevity Research, in which enzymes were praised for their ability to combat cancer. It said that enzymes deter the cancer cell's ability to hide from the immune system, which may thereby allow the cells to spread throughout the body undetected. So, with the important involvement in every body function, it is necessary that we intake adequate enzymes on a daily basis."

"I see," her father said, nodding with comprehension.

"However, because we're not cows or rabbits," she continued, smiling at him "we can't eat wheatgrass as a food. The cellulose content is too high for us to assimilate with only one stomach, so we need to juice it. By drinking one ounce of fresh wheatgrass juice, which has the equivalent nutrient value of one kilogram of green leafy vegetables *and* provides additional enzyme intake, you can feel a difference in energy, strength and endurance, and you may also experience an overall sense of well-being in your health and spirituality."

"Wow, that's impressive. So, I'll be juicing grass as well as other vegetables," her father said, "can I use the grass outside or do we have to grow this special wheat grass, and, has it been used before?"

"It's almost fifty years ago that Dr Ann Wigmore discovered that all grasses have high nutrient value due to the high chlorophyll content, and that it's just as good for humans as it is for animals," Ariena replied. "However, she also discovered that the grass produced from wheat has a higher content of all nutrients and enzymes than the other grasses, which makes it more alkaline, and therefore more palatable to humans. Chlorophyll can be extracted from many plants, but wheatgrass is superior because it has been found to have over 100 elements needed by humans. It makes up over 70 per cent of the solid content of wheatgrass juice and is therefore one of the best sources of living chlorophyll available. Since then, growing and juicing of wheatgrass has been a mainstay of the therapy she developed in healing cancer and other supposedly incurable dis-ease in the body."

"Wasn't it some years ago that a Dr Hans Fischer and a group of associates won the Nobel Prize for their work on red blood cells, where during their research, the scientists noticed that human blood, is practically identical to chlorophyll on the molecular level?" Joy commented.

"I remember that, dear," her grandmother said, "and there was a double blind study done back In 1936, where all the subjects had less than half the normal haemoglobin count," she added, "half were fed various types of chlorophyll and the others did not receive any chlorophyll. Those receiving raw, unrefined chlorophyll were able to increase the speed of haemoglobin regeneration by more than 50 per cent above average in about two weeks, but the group who did not receive chlorophyll, did not improve the speed of haemoglobin regeneration. It was concluded that the body is capable of converting raw, unrefined chlorophyll to haemoglobin."

"What exactly is chlorophyll?"

"It's the green pigment found in plants, Gramps. The leaves of the plant convert light into energy that is stored in the plant fibres. Most green plants are characterised by chlorophyll, which has magnesium as its nucleus," his granddaughter explained, drawing on her biology studies. "In the human body," she continued, "red blood cells are characterised by the oxygen carrier haemoglobin, which has as its central nucleus the mineral element iron. Since chlorophyll and haemoglobin are so much alike in atom structure, chlorophyll is absorbed quickly into the blood stream and immediately begins to rebuild blood cells. An increase of red blood cells would result in better circulation, rapid body cleansing and oxygenation to the cells. Liquid chlorophyll gets into the tissues, refines them and rebuilds them."

"Is this scientifically proven?"

"Oh, yes," Joy replied. "Science has proven that chlorophyll arrests growth and development of unfriendly bacteria, it helps purify the liver, neutralises toxins, and washes drug deposits from the body," she replied. "Oxygen is quickly used up in the many body functions that it is responsible for during infusion into the blood. Chlorophyll in wheatgrass juice stimulates an improvement in the immune system, which is our natural means of preventing and healing all kinds of illness."

"In other words," Ariena picked up the thread of the conversation, "the blood becomes richer and the body healthier by its use. Chlorophyll is the basis of all plant life, it is the first product of light and therefore contains more light energy than any other element. It was the famous Swiss physician Dr Max Bircher who said that chlorophyll is condensed solar energy."

"Is that who invented Bircher muesli?"

"Yes, it is, he also used raw food and wheatgrass juice to heal his patients."

"So, muesli is okay to have for breakfast then?"

"Sure, Gramps, so long as it's Bircher muesli, because it's raw, not cooked or processed."

"Oh, but then I can't have milk on cereal." He thought for a moment then said, "I could use orange juice instead, I suppose."

"Sure, that would probably taste quite good, but you can also make milk out of almonds."

"How do you do that? I can't imagine squeezing much out of a nut!"

"It's easy, Grandpa. You just soak the almonds overnight, rinse them off in the morning, blend them up with a little water and pour the milk through a sieve, done in 5 minutes!"

"Does sound easy, I'll try it," he said enthusiastically, "cos I do like my cereal for breakfast."

"You know, it was Dr Bircher who said that it's the very same power that enables clumps of grass to push their way through cement sidewalks in a matter of days, that is available to our bodies, through drinking wheatgrass juice."

"Good old Dr Bircher, he knew a thing or two, if he says we should have wheatgrass juice, then we'll have it!" Ariena smiled at her father's resolve.

"We'll have to start growing it Dad," Glen suggested, "with the amount that we'll all need. Maybe you can help me with that."

"Sure, son, I've got a green thumb when it comes to growing things. How do we grow it?"

"I've been reading up on that since Ariena mentioned it a few days ago, seems like it's not difficult," Glen replied. "We just need a few trays, some organic soil, water and good ventilation. It's very quick to grow too," he added, "only a week and you can start harvesting it, but while we're waiting for the first lot to grow, you'd better start juicing the lawn, since we wont have time to mow it!"

"Okay, Nana and I will go in tomorrow and buy a juicer, so we can get right on it!"

"Great, if you also get some organic wheat seeds while you're there and I'll get the soil and trays, we can get started on growing the grass tomorrow as well."

"Sounds like you two are starting a grow-op Gramps," Scott said.

"It's not that kind of grass, young man," his grandfather replied, "this here wheatgrass is *real* medicine!"

Ariena burst out laughing. "You're absolutely right Dad," she said with a chuckle, "it was Dr Ann Wigmore who said that wheatgrass is nature's *finest* medicine."

# CHAPTER 12
# HOPE

Ariena reached the top of the stairs and took in the scene before her. A crowd of women were waiting to enter the room. Some stood in small groups chatting easily together while others stood by themselves. Two women carrying a box so large, Ariena could hardly see their faces were puffing their way up the stairs. As they reached the top step, they both dropped the box in front of them.

"Hi everyone," the woman standing nearest to Ariena called out, "sorry we're late, we need a lift in this building!" She pulled a key out of her coat pocket and walked across the landing towards the door.

"Come on in," she called as she unlocked the door.

"Can I carry the boxes in?" Ariena asked, stepping forward. She didn't wait for an answer, as she put one box on top of the other and lifted both.

"Wow, you're stronger than you look," commented the woman at the door, "can you take them all the way to the front please." The other women filed into the room and started seating themselves.

"Can everybody please use the chairs up front," the woman with the keys called out as she bustled past, "that way if anyone comes late they can pop into the back seats without interrupting the meeting," she said, as she settled herself into one of two chairs set behind a table at the front of the room.

Ariena put the boxes beside the table and sat in the front row. Within five minutes everyone was seated and an air of excitement drifted through the room. The two women seated behind the table stood up. "Thanks for coming everyone, this is a momentous occasion! It's been a few months since we decided to get a group together in our community, and it is wonderful to see so many here this evening. We're all here for the same reason, to support each other in our journey with cancer. In one way we're all the same, we've all been diagnosed with cancer and are going through various stages of living with cancer, but in many ways we are all different. Our diagnoses are different, our treatments and therapies are different, our ages and personal lives are different, no doubt we think differently, and obviously, those of us who are taking tamoxifin know that our sizes are different!" Laughter erupted in the room.

"We're here this evening to form a support group that will come together using the strength of all our differences, to support each other in our common goal to survive!" All the women cheered enthusiastically.

"We're already survivors!" someone called out.

"Yes, indeed we are, but we are survivors with a purpose. We're here to support each other in a way that will bring health and happiness, and above all, *hope* into our lives. We're here to be a part of the best support team ever!" The women clapped and cheered loudly. As they quietened down, Ariena looked around the room, smiling broadly as she saw the excitement on the faces around her.

"This day will go down in our list of dates that we will always remember. Tonight we form our very own Dragon Boat Team, and being a cancer survivor is the only prerequisite to join!" Ariena could feel the excitement building in herself as everyone cheered again.

"As I said before, we are all different. We all have our own strengths and weaknesses, but as a Cancer Survivor Team, we will use those attributes to our collective advantage. This evening we can *all* sign on to be a part of the Team, there is no reason for any of us not to join, there will be a place on the Team for each of us. Now, as I pointed out earlier, some of us are obviously less physically fit than others, but we can all pull our weight in some way, so to speak." Ariena smiled at the play on words. "There's more to this Team than the sport aspect of it. Certainly, dragon boating is a physically demanding sport, but I'm sure we will learn the techniques and train to compete in the sport to the best of our physical abilities, and that is all we can expect of each other. However, the most important aspect of this Team, is the emotional and mental support we can share with one another. We all know how hard it is to live with the stress that comes with cancer. We all know how hard it is to be positive sometimes, how hard it is to get through a bad day. We all know how it feels to have doubts and how often we think that fear will completely consume us. We all know the utter despair of feeling completely alone, and it's all we can do to stay afloat in a sea of hopelessness."

The speaker's voice caught in her throat. She sat down, unable to continue. The woman next to her reached over and gave her a hug. There was not a dry eye in the room. Ariena turned to the woman sitting next to her and reached out to give her a hug. The quiet sound of muffled sobs intermingled with timid laughter, as everyone in the room followed suit. Finally, as the emotion in the room dissipated, the speaker stood up and continued.

"Forming a Dragon Boat Team amongst cancer survivors is all about forming a bond to support each other on our physical, emotional and even spiritual journey, and above all else, to keep hope afloat!" A cheer went up and everyone stood, clapping and hugging each other while introducing themselves, as the wave of excitement reentered the room.

"Okay, everyone, now that we're all acquainted, let's get down to business!"

A hum of anticipation filled the room as they all returned to their seats. The speaker placed several sheets of paper and a pile of pens on the table in front of her. "Everyone is welcome to sign up to join the Team now," she announced as she stepped forward to open the two boxes. She reached in to one and pulled out a life jacket and from the other box she took out a long wooden paddle. Holding both her arms high, so everyone could see, she said, "Please sign your name beside a number on the sheet, and then you can come and take a paddle and a life jacket with your corresponding number. They will be yours for as long as you are in the Team, and now, since we're all in the same boat, so to speak, let's have tea and cake, and get to know our fellow team members." The room filled with the sound of laughter and clapping, a room full of women brought together by a common need for support on their journey of hope.

*

"Okay Team, listen up," Ariena called out, as she walked across the grass and stopped in front of the large group of women, "the Committee has asked me to show you some exercises we can be doing as a training routine before and after practice."

"Hope it's going to warm us up, it's freezing this morning!"

"It will do that, and it will help with our overall fitness," Ariena replied. "Even though we're a recreational team, we are going to be competing in the annual dragon boat festival next month, so we might as well give it all we've got!"

"That's okay for you, you're an athlete! It's all the rest of us can do to just get in the boat, let alone paddle. Now you want us to exercise as well? We're not in any shape to exercise!"

"That's the point I think," Ariena replied, "if you start exercising, you will get fitter, stronger and healthier. It doesn't matter what shape you're in now, everyone can do some gentle exercise daily that will make a huge difference. Exercise is one of the best ways of enhancing your body's elimination functions. Just 15 minutes of gentle exercise each day can heighten your sense of well-being and enhance your self-esteem. It can enhance creativity and improve your outlook on life, increase your IQ and improve the memory."

"I think most of us need that, the old chemo brain doesn't work so good any more."

"Well," Ariena continued, "regular exercise will improve concentration and increase mental sharpness, it will release anxiety and depression. They say, the more you exercise the longer your life!"

"Exercise makes me sleep!"

"Really, it wakens me up!"

"Either way, it's good," Ariena laughed, "regular exercise will help you to have a deeper sleep, but if you can't get to sleep, I've heard it improves your sexual performance!"

"Now you're talking!" Everyone laughed.

\*

"You can build up your level of activity and improve your overall fitness slowly," Ariena continued, "exercise is too often promoted to burn fat and lose weight, rather than for its health inducing aspects. The simplest way to increase your daily exercise is to walk. Walk to and from work if possible, if not, take a walk in the park at lunchtime or after work. Walk up and down stairs instead of taking the lift and in the evenings take a stroll along the beach or in the park. Alternatively, go for a bike ride or go for a swim, or of course, you can go for a run!"

"No, we'll leave the running to you!"

Ariena smiled. "I will show you a couple of exercise routines today that include gentle stretching exercises, which are very simple and effective. You can also do them at home or get together with your paddling partner and make up your own workout sessions," she continued, "but don't overdo it, let the body stretch and bend naturally and each time you do the exercises you will find you can do just a little more. The key is to keep within your own capabilities, but to never stop pushing, just enough to take you to the next level of fitness."

"Okay, we're game to try, but what about the days when we're not coming here for practice, how are our chemo brains going to remember the routine at home?"

Everyone laughed at the inside joke.

"Don't worry, I've written it out and there's a copy for each of you to take home," she replied, "and I've also got a surprise for you after today's practice."

"Hope you're not going to expect us to take up running as well, are you?"

"Not unless you want to," Ariena replied with a laugh, "no, I'll do the running, but there is something else that we can be doing on a regular basis that will help us in competition, but I'll tell you about it after practice."

*

Ariena skillfully steered the boat alongside the dock, passing the rope to the paddler sitting in front of where she was standing at the stern. With the boat securely tied up, she jumped ashore and held the hull steady for the others to get out. The women milled about on the dock, taking their teammate's paddles as they alighted, bailing water from the boat and chatting about the day's practice.

"So, what's the surprise you've got for us?" someone called out to Ariena. She checked again that the boat was secure and stood up.

"You're all invited to come down to our restaurant and have an energy lunch!" she announced.

*

When everyone had arrived at the Health Centre that Ariena and Glen had established the year after she had been diagnosed with cancer, she showed them through to the private function area in the restaurant.

"I've told the girls we'll be having lunch in here, so we wont be disturbed," she explained.

"The Health Centre is wonderful, and the restaurant is lovely, you've done a great job Ariena," one of her Team mates commented as they walked through.

"Wait till you taste the food, it's delicious!" another said enthusiastically.

"Yes, *and* healthy! It's great to have a healthy option."

"I heard your health talks are going well Ariena, you've had some famous health educators speak here."

"Did you attend the festival she put on? It went on for ten days, with speakers from all over. I went to some of the talks and activities, it was great!"

"I read in the paper that you offer personalised health programs now."

"*And* there's a fitness room and spa with an infrared sauna!"

Ariena put her hands up. "Whoa, thanks everyone," she said with a laugh, "and yes, we do offer health programs, and the health talks are ongoing in the conference hall at the back of the restaurant. There are a lot of things going on in the Centre," she added, "and that is why I invited you all here today. Apart from having lunch together, I'd like to offer everyone on the Team the opportunity to make use of our facilities here. Today's lunch is on the house," she continued, "so you can try the different juices and raw vegan food that is on the menu." The women clapped and cheered.

"As you know," she continued, "this Centre has come into being as a result of my own healing journey with cancer. We wanted to create a place where we could share the knowledge and experience we have gained through the conscious lifestyle choices I made, after I received my diagnosis. We share the information through our talks, the lifestyle programs, classes and presentations we give at the Centre," she explained, "and we share the passion we have for the healthy diet and fitness regime, that has made such a difference in my life, here in the restaurant and in the spa."

The women sat around the table listening intently.

"Joining our dragon boat team has been one of the best decisions I have made in my journey back to health," Ariena continued, smiling at the nods of agreement, "and it continues to play an essential part of my ongoing healing. The comradeship, the team spirit and the friendship that each of you provide in my life is of great value to me." She smiled as the women nodded at each other. "I know that you all feel the same way," she went on, "we are a very special group, that not only provides support for each other, but we really do keep hope afloat!"

Everyone clapped spontaneously.

Ariena smiled at her friends. "So, because you're all so special," she said, "I would like to give every member of the Team a special membership to our Centre and discounts in the restaurant and store. You are all welcome to attend the health talks and events we put on here, and you can come in to use the fitness room or have an infrared sauna in the spa anytime, just phone ahead for an appointment," she laughed.

"Wow, that's fantastic, thank you so much," one of the women said as they all clapped again.

"I'd love to hear what you did to get so fit and healthy," another commented.

"Well, I can share a little about raw nutrition while we eat lunch today," Ariena replied, "and I can certainly give you lots of fitness *and* relaxation tips."

"What we need to know is how to increase and maintain our energy levels, so we can win that race next month!"

*

Amid appreciative chatter, platters of delicious looking food was brought to the table, and in front of each person, a small shot glass was placed. A deep emerald green liquid sparkled through the glass. "What is this?"

Ariena stood up and raised her shot glass. "This, my friends," she said, "is wheatgrass juice, Nature's finest medicine! This beautiful green liquid holds all the secrets to our success!" she added dramatically, catching everyone's attention.

"We're going to be drinking grass?"

"All this food looks absolutely delicious, even if it isn't cooked, but I don't know about drinking grass!"

"I thought your juices were made from vegetables and fruit, no-one said anything about grass!"

"Well, ladies," Ariena replied with a smile, "if you want to increase your energy levels, this will do it! Eating more raw fruit and vegetables and drinking fresh juice will do the same, but over a longer period of time. Wheatgrass juice will give you instant energy, and at the same time, it will help the body to kick into detoxing, which we all need to do constantly."

"Oh, dear. I don't like the sound of this, detoxing you say?"

"*Energy*, I said," Ariena replied, "instant energy! Don't worry about the detoxing, I'll tell you all about how that works later. Just focus on the raw energy!" She lifted the shot glass again to regain their attention. "Wheatgrass juice is a complete food, it has all the nutrients you need, not only to survive, but to thrive!" she said, "surviving is what we're doing now, but thriving is what we really want to do!"

"Hear, hear!"

"Now, I should warn you," she said with a smile, "the taste of wheatgrass juice is, shall we say, a little interesting. That is because wheatgrass is pure alkaline, so if your body is more on the acidic side, it will taste a little bitter. However, when you include more alkaline foods in your diet, such as fresh fruits and vegetables and raw vegan foods, your body will become more alkaline, and the wheatgrass will taste sweet. It's a good way to gauge how your pH level is, have a shot of wheatgrass every day!"

"Sounds scary, can we have something to chase it?"

"It's best taken on it's own," Ariena replied, "that way it can quickly enter the bloodstream and the body can assimilate the nutrients. However, if you really need to, you can have a mouthful of the fresh carrot juice," she said, pointing to the jug of brilliant orange coloured juice on the table. "It's also best to swish the wheatgrass juice around you mouth before swallowing it," she continued, "so it mixes with the saliva and enzymes in your mouth. That makes it even easier for the body to assimilate the nutrients, and it usually tastes better if you do that than just downing the shot." She lifted her glass and demonstrated. "Mmm, delicious," she said, watching with amusement as everyone followed suit. She reached for the jug of carrot juice and started pouring it into their glasses. "You'll get used to it," she said with a laugh, as several took a gulp of carrot juice, "and I promise it will get sweeter as you get healthier. From now on, I'll bring some down to every practice, so you can all get that extra energy we need when we're paddling."

"Oh, dear, this is a bit extreme isn't it?"

"I find it quite sweet, I must be more alkaline than I thought."

"Me too, I guess it depends on what you've been eating the day before."

"Yes, and what you're stress level is, that's acid forming in the body too."

"When you think about it, drinking wheatgrass juice is the same as the cow and other animals eating grass, and they are all living on it so it must be loaded with enough nutrients to keep them healthy."

"Exactly," Ariena agreed, "so drinking wheatgrass juice and eating raw fruit and vegetables is not really extreme at all. As a vegan, I think it's more extreme to eat the cow."

"Hmm, I'll have to think on that."

"Good idea, thinking consciously has certainly improved my health," Ariena replied.

"Yes, it's obvious. Please, do tell us about it."

\*

"Eating nutritious foods and regular exercise are two of the most important factors for overall health. Nutritious foods provide fuel to the body while exercise raises the metabolism, which converts the fuel to energy, and without energy, movement of the body becomes difficult," Ariena began. "Put it this way," she continued, "as with a car, the body is designed to move. It is our first form of transportation. The body is an incredible machine which, when fuelled and run correctly, will keep ticking over at a healthy rate for many years. We all know that without the right type of fuel, a car will not run smoothly, and with no fuel to burn, the car will be running on empty. Without lubrication, the parts of the motor will not be able to move and will need replacing, or they will eventually cease up, and the car will stop running. It is the same with the human body. The wrong fuel is exactly what the average diet is made up of, acid forming foods such as meat, eggs, dairy, alcohol, and grains, especially wheat. Diets high in such foods put a great strain on the digestive system and deplete the body's energy levels. Our bodies need alkaline, or clean burning food, such as fresh, nutritious, raw fruits, vegetables and juices to act as fuel and give us energy. Regular exercise raises the metabolism to ensure a healthy body and a healthy lifestyle to keep the heart, which is our motor, and organs operating efficiently. The body will not stop running as a result."

"If eating raw food is as good as this, I'm going to try it, this is all so delicious! Can we have the recipes?"

Ariena laughed. "Best to keep it simple for now," she suggested, "just start by including more fresh raw fruit and veggies in your diet, and you can come in here for the special dishes."

"I've tried so many diets, but none of them have food like this. They are so complicated and they don't work, so I end up fat *and* depressed. Sometimes I feel like I'm never going to win! I guess if I eat fruit and vegetables it will be a healthy way to lose weight, and easy too."

"Yes," Ariena agreed, "most conventional slimming or weight loss diets have strict regimes of calorie-counted, portion-controlled meals, and strenuous fat-burning exercises. They very rarely, if at all, take into account that our emotions and physical well-being are linked. Those diets most often fail because they do not take into account that the body is the vehicle that carries these feelings and that the mind is the engine that drives and motivates the body. Everything is linked."

"Well, since we're more likely to be emotionally motivated, we'd better get it right! So, how does the diet and fitness link to give us the energy we need to win that race?"

\*

"Getting fit and raising your metabolism will raise your energy level and enhance a healthy lifestyle," Ariena replied, "by starting your race towards optimal health, you have the chance to win. So, this is not just about the race next month, it's about the race for life!"

"Here, here!"

"A regular exercise program will provide oxygen to the blood and therefore help to increase blood circulation," Ariena continued, "physical activity will make the heart stronger, it strengthens the organs, increases muscle tone, decreases blood cholesterol, reduces tension and burns more calories."

"Oh, no, not calories, we're not going to be counting calories are we?"

"It is not necessary to count calories if the diet is based on healthy foods that provide the necessary nutrients and live enzymes needed by the body," Ariena replied, "a calorie is a unit used to measure energy, and for optimal health, your calorie intake should reflect your exercise level. If your intake is high, your exercise level should increase, to ensure a higher metabolism, thereby converting the fuel into energy."

"Phew! Thank goodness for that! I'm all for keeping it simple."

"You're saying that if we just eat fruits and vegetables and do some exercise, we'll be healthy and have lots of energy? Surely, it can't be that simple."

"Being healthy and energetic really is that simple," Ariena replied, "you see, the body gets energy primarily from three sources, carbohydrates, fat and protein. Not only does plant food supply all these fuels, but a fit and healthy body can also convert its own stores into energy. Most of the calories should come from usable carbohydrates such fresh fruit and vegetables and good fats are found in avocados, nuts and seeds."

"What about your protein? If you're only eating fruits and vegetables, where do you get your protein?" Ariena smiled. "Same place the cow gets it," she replied, "from the grass!"

"You mean the wheatgrass juice?"

"Yep, exactly," Ariena replied, "all grass and fresh greens are rich in protein. Like I said, that's where the animals get their protein from. I do too, I just don't pass it through the cow first!"

"Wow, I never thought of that."

"No, most people don't," Ariena said, "that's because we've been led to believe that eggs, fish, meat and dairy products are the only source of protein, but clearly that is not true. The truth is that animal foods provide excessive amounts of protein as well as saturated fats, which lead to ill health in humans. Many medical studies now show that consuming meat, dairy and other animal products, cause serious ill health, such as heart disease, diabetes, *and* cancer. Believe me," she added, "you can get all the nutrients you need from a healthy, well balanced plant-based diet."

"Well, you're living proof of that!"

"Yes," Ariena agreed, "and I intend to stay that way! I'm going to live my life, not spend it dying, and when my time comes," she added with a smile, "I'm going out mid air!"

Everyone cheered. "Well said, we're with you all the way, girl!"

"Good, I'm glad to hear it!" Ariena replied. "Remember, we're all in the same boat, so let's keep our paddles up and do everything we can to be fit and healthy!" The women clapped spontaneously again, all nodding in agreement with what Ariena had said.

"Thank you so much for inviting us here, for the wonderful lunch and for all the health tips you've shared. The food is delicious, we all think you should write a recipe book!"

"Perhaps I will one day," Ariena smiled, "but meanwhile, I'm happy to share what I know. Before you leave, I'll show you all around the fitness room and infrared sauna spa, so you can come in and make use of the facilities as often as you want."

"Yay! Now you're talking. All this exercising and eating, we were wondering when we get to do the relaxing!"

"There are many simple and effective daily gentle exercises designed to boost your energy levels *and* to relax effectively," Ariena replied with a laugh, "and there are several methods of improving your energy flow to balance your body *and* mind. Some of the things you can do include simple yoga exercises, take a relaxing bath, have massage and reflexology sessions, as well as practicing conscious relaxation."

"With all that going on, we wont have time to breathe!"

"Interesting you should say that," Ariena said, "breathing is a reflex action that the body does automatically without any help from us consciously doing it. This reflex action helps the oxygen to flow around the body to all the vital organs, and if we practice breathing in and out in a deep controlled way, it not only increases the amount of oxygen supplied to the blood, but it is also a relaxing way to center ourselves. The more the body is filled with oxygen through deep breathing, the less stress you place on the body and subsequently, the mind," she explained. "The more you consciously practice deep, controlled breathing, the more natural it becomes and you can use it any time of day to help you through tired and stressful moments. If you think about the very act of breathing bringing in a life-giving force to your body, you will consciously feel its energy flowing through you and healing you."

"That's very true, every time I take a deep breath, it has a very cleansing feeling."

"You're right, together with the alkaline foods you eat, and the fresh juices and water you drink, conscious breathing will gently cleanse your body from the inside," Ariena said, "but it is also important to cleanse the outside of the body. As our bodies become cleansed, so do our minds, and with regular practice, you can build up a store of physical and mental energy that you can draw on whenever you need to."

"Like during the race next month!"

"Exactly, literally anytime you need to, the body stores energy for when you most need it."

"Tell us about yoga, do you have classes here?"

"Yoga consists of physical exercises and breathing practices for achieving and maintaining bodily health and fitness, *and* to still the mind by concentrating on our energies," she replied. "It is possibly the best exercise you can do, because it combines meditation with physical fitness to ensure that the mind and body function efficiently and to their maximum potential. Several of our associated practitioners are yoga teachers, and there are two yoga studios in town I would highly recommend you join if you haven't done it before."

"So what are the methods of relaxing that we can do at home?"

"Well, I'm sure everyone here enjoys a bath," Ariena replied, "I've heard it said, 'never get between a woman and her bath' so go ahead and take over the bathroom whenever you can, but at least once a week, plan to have a bath in the evening, so you can enjoy it. Run a deep bath at a comfortable warm temperature and pour in about 2 cups of Epsom salts, stirring until it is dissolved."

"What's Epsom salts? Are they different to bath salts?"

"Yes," Ariena replied, "most bath salts are regular just salt with colouring and perfume added, usually chemical based and therefore toxic, not what I would recommend bathing in. Epsom salts are pure magnesium crystals that are vital for the body's cellular activity, they speed up the circulation and draw toxins from the body," she explained. "Just relax for about five minutes in the bath to soften the skin, then using a loofah or massage mitt, massage the body using gentle strokes along the limbs towards the heart. Lie back and relax for another 10 minutes. Towel dry and wrap up warm, then sit or lie down for an hour, play some soft music and relax. As you will feel quite warm and relaxed afterward, you will also enjoy a great sleep without interruption."

"I like to have a scented bath, so if you can't use bath salts, do Epsom salts have a scent?"

"No, and there is no added perfume when you get pure Epsom salts. The easiest way to add natural scent to your bath is with herbs and therapeutic oils. Put a small quantity of fresh or dried herbs in a muslin bag and hang it from the tap so the warm water flows through and releases the aromatic oils naturally. Essential and aromatherapy oils are well known for their beneficial properties, and depending on the oils or herbs that are added to the water, baths can be either relaxing or invigorating."

"What are some of the herbs you can use?"

"Well, for relaxing herbal baths, you could use chamomile, jasmine, valerian, meadowsweet, lime flowers and lavender. For stimulating herbal baths, choose from basil, bay, eucalyptus, fennel, lemon balm and lemon verbena, mint, pine, rosemary, sage and thyme."

"Sounds like a song, parsley, sage, rosemary and thyme. Is parsley good for cleansing too?"

"Yes, especially when you eat it!"

"I heard that you have to be careful using essential oils, because they are so concentrated."

"That's true," Ariena agreed, "the safest way to start using essential or aromatherapy oils is to buy ready prepared natural blends, but always read the ingredient list. All essential oils and aromatherapy massage oils, must be diluted in a carrier oil, such as almond oil, or dispersed into a medium such as bath water. Essential or aromatherapy oils can also be released into the atmosphere with an oil burner," she added, "I like to have an Epsom salt bath with a candle lit and my favourite essential oil wafting in the air, a relaxing bath is all about the ambiance!"

"What's your recommendation for dry skin? My elbows and knees and my heels are the worst, but even on my arms and legs, the skin is dry and flaky."

"Exfoliating once a week is a great way to remove dead skin cells and to soften areas of hard skin around the heels or elbows and knees," Ariena replied, "exfoliation requires water along with an exfoliating gel which you can easily make with fresh herbs, some celtic sea salt, a little almond oil and a drop or two of essential oils for aromatherapy. First you relax in a warm bath for 10 minutes to allow the skin to soften," she continued, "then you apply a small amount of exfoliating scrub with gentle circular stokes all over the body, especially around the feet, elbows and knees. Re-immerse yourself in the water and continue with the circular movements until the scrub is washed away, taking all the dead cells with it!"

"What if you don't have a bath, we've only got a shower."

"Dry skin brushing is a simple process that not only improves the quality of your skin by removing dead skin cells, but it also stimulates the body's production of sebum, a natural oily secretion of the sebaceous glands, which moisturises the skin. It is also an excellent method of improving blood circulation and improved lymph flow, which means more efficient elimination of toxins and wastes in the body, *and* it encourages new cell growth."

"So, you mean, you brush yourself with a dry brush?"

"Yes, exactly," Ariena replied, "you don't wet the brush or the skin. Dry brushing is quick and convenient because it does not require anything more than a few minutes each morning using a long handled brush or a loofah. Just spend a couple of minutes dry brushing all parts of the body. Starting at the feet, stroke upwards and toward the heart, using several long firm strokes on the feet, legs, buttocks and back. Use very gentle circular strokes in a clockwise direction on the delicate stomach area, and don't brush the breasts."

"Don't need to worry, I haven't got any."

Ariena smiled, "Then you don't need to worry either," she said. "Keep brushing the arms from wrist to shoulder, up the back of neck to the base of the skull. You can brush your face as well, but use a soft, dry face cloth or special facial brush."

"Okay, that sounds good, any tips for when I'm in the shower?"

"Yes, sing!"

"Oh, I do that already, always ensures I get the bathroom to myself!"

"Good one," Ariena laughed, "but after your regular shower in the morning, turn the water to cold for a minute. The cold water firms up the skin and improves muscle tone while awakening your body and mind."

"Are you kidding? I get in the shower to get warm!"

"Yes, but this leaves you feeling even warmer, because the cold water increases the circulation," she replied, "and when you're washing your face, splash with cold water afterwards to tone and tighten the skin. You'll see, it's really great!" Ariena smiled encouragingly. "You know," she said kindly, "something else you can do that is wonderful for the soul, is to take a cool swim in the sea or paddle barefoot up to your ankles for a few minutes, it's very refreshing."

"Did you hear that girls? Next practice we throw her in!"

Ariena burst out laughing, "You'll have to catch me first," she said, "but really, being in cold water is so invigorating, I wouldn't mind. I love running in the rain, it cools me down."

"I don't know, next you'll be wanting us to go stand in the rain!"

"I think, an even better idea, would be to dance in the rain!" Everyone laughed at their friendly banter. "You mentioned reflexology, I've heard of it, but I've never tried it."

"Reflexology is a therapy that dates as far back as ancient Egypt and is based on the idea that there are reflex points, or zones on the feet, which relate to points, organs and systems in the body," Ariena replied. "By working these points or zones on the feet, reflexologists can relieve imbalances or illnesses in the corresponding points in the body. When you have a complete treatment with a professional therapist, they can give you tips on how to do your own reflexology on yourself or with a friend."

"Maybe we should get a group booking."

"That's a great idea. I'll see if I can arrange it."

"Can you arrange for us all to have a massage too?"

Ariena chuckled. "That might be a little difficult, but I've heard that there will be massage therapists at the dragon boat festival, so don't forget to line up! Some of us could have a massage before the race to release tension and relax the mind, while some of us can have it afterwards, to lower the heart rate and relieve muscle soreness."

"Great idea!"

"Massage is also one of the oldest and natural types of therapy known," Ariena continued, "and as it is designed to improve circulation and skin tone, while relaxing the body, it also helps the efficient flow of lymph through the lymphatic system, something we all need to be aware of. So, a little self-massage would be good before the race, to keep those arms and paddles moving!"

"Well, we all better get moving now, thank you again for all the great tips."

"They are all easy and effective methods of getting back in touch with your body," Ariena replied, "if you try to incorporate them in your everyday life, along with using visualisation and saying affirmations, it will all nourish the body and the spirit."

"My biggest problem is memory, the old chemo brain is not going to remember it all!"

Ariena smiled. "Don't worry, I've got a tip list for everyone, so there's no excuses!" she replied, "There's only 20 things to remember, I'll quickly read them out and you can take one when you go."

*

1. Drink a large glass of warm water with lemon juice first thing each morning.
2. Increase your intake of fresh raw fruit and vegetables, by eating, and/or juicing at least three portions of vegetables per day, or juice your veggies and use the juice to make delicious energy soups.
3. Eat three portions of fruit and three portions of salad per day.
4. Remember that you are not restricted to portion size. You should feel satisfied with the quantities, quality and variety of the foods you eat. Fibre is provided by fresh fruit and vegetables and raw juices, which is a soluble and gentle cleanser of the intestines, especially the colon. Commonly used fibre such as wheat bran or powders, are insoluble,

difficult to digest and harsh on the body, so are therefore not recommended.

5. Remember you can snack between meals so prepare some goodie bags with raw carrot sticks or mixed nuts and seeds.

6. Eat 12 soaked almonds per day.

7. Have one tablespoon of freshly ground flaxseed every day, add to juices, soups or sprinkle on salads.

8. Increase your good fluid intake, drink at least 2 litres of fluid every day, including raw juices, pure water and herbal teas. Juices are a highly concentrated source of unprocessed, natural, alkaline forming, and enzyme-rich nutrition. Freshly made wheatgrass juice and raw vegetable juices are vital, because they are both highly alkaline forming and are packed full of antioxidants and live enzymes. Drinking pure water cleanses and eliminates the accumulated toxins within and keeps each of the vital organs working efficiently. The minimum amount of fluids required by the body each day is 6-8 glasses, to replace what is lost naturally.

9. Exercise for at least 30 minutes each day, start out gently to include 15 minutes of stretching. Do yoga at home or take yoga classes, and walk instead of driving when possible.

10. Take 5 minutes every day to do your conscious deep breathing.

11. Dry brush your skin every morning.

12. Take a cold shower or splash yourself with cold water every morning.

13. Do a self massage every day, it only takes a few minutes!

14. Every 3 days, exfoliate!

15. Every 5 days, take an Epsom salts bath.

16. Whenever you can, treat yourself to a professional body therapy – a massage aromatherapy or reflexology.

17.  Say your affirmations 10 times throughout the day.
18.  Eliminate coffee, tea and soft drinks. All drinks that contain caffeine and sugars are highly addictive and can therefore be difficult to give up immediately. You can break the habit slowly, with the goal of eliminating it entirely, by using a smaller cup and immediately reducing your daily intake by at least half.
19.  Decrease and eventually eliminate all meats, dairy products, eggs and fish, processed and junk foods, hydrogenated fats and oils, refined foods especially white sugar and flour, salt, fried foods, grilled, barbequed or burnt foods, all commercially prepared fruit and vegetables, all grains especially wheat, non organic dried fruits, rhubarb, peanuts, coffee, tea, hot chocolate and malted drinks, carbonated water and soft drinks, canned and boxed juices, alcohol, nicotine and all drugs.
20.  Quit smoking – no excuses, just do it!

*

Ariena arrived at the Team tent half an hour before the race. Everyone gathered round as she opened the ice box. "There's enough for a double shot each," she said, as she lifted the jug filled with bright green liquid. She handed a stack of shot glasses to one of the women, who took one and passed them on. Ariena poured the wheatgrass juice into each shot glass as they filed past. When everyone had a full glass, Ariena held hers up. "To our absent teammates," she said.

"To Team Spirits!"

"To keeping hope afloat!"

"Paddles Up!"

\*

Tension was building as all paddles held still beside the hull. Ariena loosened her grip on the tiller, stretched her fingers and closed them tightly over the smooth wood. The boat sat dead in the water, prow pointing in the direction of the inner harbour. Ariena could see the brightly coloured flags fluttering in the breeze, marking the finish line. She looked up the length of the boat, every head was down, every foot braced against the seat in front, every hand tightly holding a paddle. She looked forward to the drummer, her hands poised above the drum. Not a sound came from anyone, the silence was deafening. The first bell rang out over the water.

"Focus!"

The second bell sounded.

"Paddles Up!"

All paddles raised in unison. The start gun cracked through the air and 120 paddles hit the water. Five boats surged forward, their teams reaching and pulling their paddles through the water, the sound of splashing hardly audible over the yelling in the boats, and the cheering from spectators on shore. As their boat surged forward, the prow lifting high above the water, Ariena braced her feet and dug her toes in to stop from being thrown back. She tightened her grip on the tiller and focussed on the boat in front.

They were closing.

She pushed the tiller slightly leeward and felt the pull of their slipstream. "Pull!" she yelled. The paddles held in unison, the strokes deeper and stronger, increasing the speed. The sound of the drum boomed to each stroke.

"Pull!" the drummer yelled, as their prow passed the stern of the boat in front. Everyone pulled harder. Ariena felt the pull of the other boat's slipstream, dragging them closer. She pulled the tiller back to a straight forward position. Silently she counted, *1, 2…* Every muscle in her body tensed. As the boats leveled out, dangerously close, she thrust the tiller over and held it firm. Every sinew in her arm screamed. "Pull!" she yelled again. She felt the boat surge forward, the prow lifting high out of the water.

"Pull!" everyone yelled.

She heard the roar of the crowd on shore, and she knew it was time. "Dig!" she yelled. She heard the boom of the drum as it picked up momentum.

"Dig!" everyone yelled. Then she felt it. An invisible power took hold of the boat and lifted her free. The tension in the tiller loosened. They surged forward, and their speed increased. The crowd roared.

Ariena looked ahead, her eyes focussing on the prow and the flags at the finish line. They were closing fast. She grit her teeth and held on.

"Dig! Dig! Dig!" She could hear the excitement, she could feel the tension, she could taste the adrenalin. She knew, the critical moment was upon them.

"Now!" she yelled. A resounding cry rose up from the boat, every paddle sliced into the water. The boat shuddered, and, for a moment everything seemed to stand still. Ariena knew that the force behind those paddles had propelled the boat clean out of the water, and In that split second, they flew. Like an eagle on the wing, they soared through the air, enveloped by the invisible power. The prow sliced back into the water, and she felt the speed arrest slightly. At the same moment all paddles sliced into the water and, with enormous effort, the paddlers pulled. The boat shot forward, and the dragon's head burst through the finish line.

"Stop the boat!"

All paddles held fast in the water. They had done it. This race, they had won.

*

The shadows of the night slowly lifted as dawn broke, and a pink glow filled the sky. The wooden blades cut deep into the water, an effervescent burst of tiny bubbles surfacing as they slid smoothly alongside the shiny hull. Cutting a silver path through the deep blue of the early morning ocean, the boat surged forward towards the dimly lit horizon. The black silhouette moved gracefully onwards seemingly propelled by an unseen force, the only sound a watery swoosh, as 24 paddles dipped and pulled in perfect unison. Ariena stood at the stern, her feet braced against the gunwales, balancing herself against the rhythmic pull of the paddles, her hand on the tiller guiding the boat forward. She kept her eye on the horizon ahead, watching for the moment when the sun would rise from the watery depths, bringing a golden hue to another day. As the morning light slowly increased, and pink faded to yellow, Ariena watched as the first ray of sunshine burst through the water, heralding a new day.

"Paddles up!" Twenty-four paddles rose together, water glistening on the blades in the brilliant sunlight. Ariena held the tiller straight as the boat drifted on, losing momentum as it slowed. She watched as the paddlers slowly lowered their paddles to cross their partner's blade. The boat drifted to a halt, the calm waters lapping gently on the hull. Then, as the sunlight danced upon the water, 24 pink roses were thrown high above the boat, and the paddlers began to sing. Their lilting voices drifting across the water, the roses floating on the surface surrounding the boat.

The paddlers' heads turned skywards as their song finished, and Ariena's heart filled with sorrow for the loss of her teammate. She raised her own head and looked skyward as a lone eagle appeared above the horizon. The giant bird flew directly towards them, it's beautifully plumed pure white head lowered. The paddlers watched as it circled above them once, swooped over the boat and then was gone.

Ariena looked beyond the paddlers to the dragon's head at the prow of the boat. She lowered her gaze and nodded. The drummer raised her arm, drumstick in hand, and brought it down on the drum with a deep resounding note. The boom bounced across the water and echoed around the bay.

"Paddles up!" Ariena called. As the women raised their paddles, the drum sounded a deep boom again. On the third beat of the drum, the wooden blades cut deep into the water and the boat propelled forward. Ariena pushed the tiller, and the boat slowly started to turn. She held the tiller fast as the prow moved across the horizon. The paddles dipped and pulled in perfect unison to the beat of the drum, the boat cutting through the circle of roses, as they bobbed away.

Ariena guided the boat in the direction of the harbour from whence they had come. She held the tiller fast as she turned and looked behind. She could no longer see the roses on the water, but in the distance, she saw a black silhouette against the sky. The eagle spread it's wings and she heard it call.

# CHAPTER 13
# TWO CHOICES

The two friends stepped out of the car, pulling their gloves on and adjusting their hats. They walked together through the parking lot, heading down towards the river. Ariena stopped and pointed up into the trees. An eagle perched high above them, it's white head turned away towards the mountain. She smiled at her friend, who nodded with a knowing smile. Neither of them spoke, they didn't need to. They both knew why the eagle was there.

*

The trail wound it's way through the trees, becoming narrower as it went deeper into the forest. They ran in single file now, Ariena leading the way. It was a quiet morning on the trail, no sound except for the wind rustling through the leaves and twigs snapping beneath their feet. As they approached the stream, Ariena slowed her pace and stopped on the wooden footbridge. Her friend stopped alongside her and put her arm around her shoulder. "Is this the place?" she asked.

"No," Ariena replied, "it's way up the mountain, in a spot where you can see the whole valley and the sea beyond."

They continued on for another 20 minutes before the trail took a turn away from the river. Ariena turned to her companion and asked, "You okay to keep going? We start climbing soon, it could take half an hour to reach the first stage."

Her friend smiled at her. "Let's go," she said. The trail widened into an open area, interspersed with rocks and blackened tree stumps. The friends ran alongside each other, with their heads down watching the trail and placing their feet carefully amongst the rocks. As they rounded a corner, Ariena's friend suddenly stopped, she was staring ahead on the trail. "Is that, a bear?" she whispered, trying to quieten the sound of her own panting.

Ariena looked ahead and laughed. "No, silly," she said, giving her friend a gentle push. "That's a tree stump!"

"Oh, yeah, you're right, phew!" she said with relief as they started running again, "but just in case, what do we do if we see a bear? You told me that you've often seen them here."

"Yes, I have," Ariena confirmed. "The first few times were a little scary, but they know me now, so they usually just ignore me. I've seen five all told, a mother with three cubs and an old boy, I think he's been around these parts for a long time, he's going white around his muzzle."

"What happened with the mother and cubs? I've heard that can be very dangerous."

"Yes, it can be, if you do the wrong thing. You just have to remember that this is their home and we're only visitors. So when you see them, slow down and stop running. Don't make any movements that might alarm them, and wait. Don't turn around and run away."

"Really?"

"Yes. They will let you know if you've been accepted as a guest. So you wait."

"Okay, in that case, you can stay in front!"

"Yep, just follow me, and enjoy the scenery. If we do see bears, it's always a blessing."

"If you say so."

"You'll see, the day you come across your first bear up here, you'll know what I mean."

"Okay, I know they are spirit animals, but I prefer eagles to bears. Anyway, I'm not as confident as you, so don't get too far ahead."

"We'll stay together, that's always a good policy when running in the mountains anyway. Just let me know if you want to slow down," Ariena said as she started to climb. The trail narrowed as they entered the forest again. Winding it's way upwards, the ground beneath their feet became damp as they gained altitude and small rivulets trickled down the rocks onto the trail.

"Be careful, it gets slippery around here," Ariena warned her friend, "there's a small stream up ahead that we have to cross as well, but we can stop and get a drink there."

"Is it okay to drink?"

"It's beautiful and fresh, it's coming from a spring further up, straight out of the mountain!" Tiny droplets of water clung to the ferns that edged the stream, and lime green moss carpeted the rocks above the stream where the sparkling stream rippled down through the trees. As it crossed the trail, the stream formed a small pool, swirling around the rocks and tumbling over the edge to continue on down the mountainside. Ariena stopped, carefully stepped over the pool and put her hand out to steady her friend as she stepped across.

"It's beautiful here," she commented, standing at the edge of the pool and looking around, "I can see why you like to run up here, it's so peaceful."

Ariena nodded, and breathed in deeply as she crouched down beside the pool. "Yes, it's one of my favourite places on the mountain," she replied, "the stream always runs crystal clear and tastes so sweet." She cupped her hands beneath the water where it trickled over the edge of a rock. Bringing them to her mouth, she drank slowly, eyes closed, savouring every drop. Her friend followed her example. "That is good," she said, "there's nothing like pure spring water, especially straight off the mountain."

Ariena nodded and stood up. "We'd better keep going before the clouds roll in," she said, "it's forecast for snow today."

"I've noticed it's getting colder as we climb," her friend said.

"With a bit of luck, there might already be snow at the top," Ariena replied, "maybe ours will be the first footprints in the snow."

"Do you still come up here when the snow is deep?"

"Oh, yes," replied Ariena enthusiastically, "it slows you down a bit, but it's so invigorating, and on a sunny day, it sparkles with rainbow coloured crystals, you'll love it!" They continued on, the trail becoming more rocky as it wound it's way up through the trees.

"These rocks are amazing, they're so big and weird how they are scattered around, not like in a rocky outcrop or anything. They look like they've dropped out of the sky!"

"They have! I thought it was strange too when I first came up here, so I did some research into the history of the area, and guess what, there was a meteor shower a few thousand years ago and apparently some fragments landed here. Some geologists did some lab tests and reckoned these rocks are from outer space!"

"Wow, that's incredible, imagine how big the meteors must have been if these are fragments, I mean, they're big rocks!"

"They are," Ariena agreed, "and there are three or four different types, most of them have lots of little indentations in them where the moss grows, but others are completely smooth and nothing grows on them at all."

So, where are yours? Are we almost there?

*

The trail wound on through the rocks and trees, climbing onward, until eventually it levelled out into an open space, a mossy rock clearing surrounded by short, stunted trees. Ariena slowed to a walk and stopped in the centre of the clearing. Her friend followed, gazing around at the perfect circle of trees and the thick carpet of moss on the ground. They looked at each other and laughed, then Ariena reached her arms up towards the sky and spun around several times. Her friend laughed again and followed suit. The two women spun around and around, until finally they collapsed on the ground, panting but still laughing and hugging each other. As their laughter ceased, a calm spread over them, and they huddled together in silence, arms wrapped around each other, their breathing becoming more shallow.

"It's beautiful," her friend eventually whispered, "it's like a zen garden, even the trees are bonsai."

"It's because of the altitude, the lack of air stunts their growth."

"How incredible, it's a natural garden, and there's a sort of ethereal presence here."

"Yes, that's universal life that you can feel. It's everywhere in nature," Ariena replied, "we're just not always aware of it, but when we immerse ourselves in nature, we become more aware and then we can sense it, feel it and sometimes even see it. Look at the trees." Her friend nodded and looked towards the trees. "It looks like there's a mist surrounding them," she said, "but it's different. It's almost like the trees are emitting the mist."

"They are," Ariena replied, "it's their energy you can see. When we are consciously connected to nature, you can see beyond what appears to be reality."

"You mean, it's like an aura?"

"Sort of, but it's pure energy. It's the life force of the tree. We have it too, all living beings do, and all animals that live in nature are connected to it, that's how they survive intuitively. Humans for the most part have lost that ability to live intuitively, to follow our instinct, like the wild animals do."

"You're right," her friend said, "we've drifted too far away from nature, and to our own detriment," she added sadly.

"That's why we have to get back to nature as much as we can," Ariena replied, hugging her friend, "so anytime you want to come up here, let me know and you can join me. I come up everyday, and every day it's different, but it gives me strength and a sense of purpose. It gives me a feeling of hope," she added, "not just for myself, but for all humankind. If we all go back to the natural way of things, there is hope that things can change. The more conscious we are of nature, the closer we will come to making real change for the better."

"Yes, and the closer we get to nature, the more we can appreciate it," her friend agreed. They sat for a while in silence, taking in the tranquil ambiance of the space.

"Do you ever feel like you're being drawn to the trees when they glow like that?"

"Oh, yes, I'm a tree hugger from way back. Do you know, if you ever feel like you need more energy, especially when you're running up the mountain, you just hug a tree and let the energy soak into you. I've done it a few times, and it really works."

"Wow, that is cool, I'll remember that."

Ariena closed her eyes and breathed in deeply several times. "Okay, I'll take you up to the cairn now," she finally said.

Stepping carefully over the moss covered rocks, Ariena entered the circle of trees. Without speaking, her friend followed. There was no trail, but Ariena knew the way well. She picked her way through the smaller rocks scattered amongst the trees, resting her hands on the larger rocks to steady herself. The twisted tree trunks were bare of leaves, and the ground covered in thick moss felt soft beneath their feet. No twigs snapped underfoot as their silent footsteps left a depression in the lush carpet. A fine mist swirled around them as they climbed higher, a dampness settled on their shoulders. Ariena looked back at her friend. "Are you okay?" she asked.

"Yes, keep going. We've come this far, I'm not stopping now."

Ariena smiled at her friend's resolve. "We're almost there," she reassured her, "just beyond this group of trees." She continued slowly, mindful of her friend's ability to keep up. Within a few minutes, she stopped, and reaching her hands out in front of her, she placed them on the huge rock. Her friend stopped behind her, then took a step to one side.

"Wow," she exclaimed, as she stared at the rock in front of her, "it's huge! Look at the depression it made on the ground, it must have come from the moon!" Then she reached her hands out and placed them on the rock too. "It feels like it's pulsating," she whispered.

Ariena smiled. "I think that's your heartbeat."

"I can feel that too, but the rock feels like it's alive."

"It is, my friend," Ariena turned and looked seriously at her, "and so are we."

Her friend looked at her sadly. "Will you build a cairn for me, Ari?" she said quietly, "then when you run up here, we'll feel each other's presence when I'm gone."

Ariena felt the whisper of a chill wind pass through her. "You're not going anywhere," she replied feebly.

Her friend turned away. "It must have taken you ages to put the smaller rocks on top," she said, changing the subject.

Ariena sighed. "One day," she replied. "I came up here on the day it was predicted I'd be dead, six months after my diagnosis. I spent all day bringing the rocks from the clearing down below, one at a time. I chose rocks that were smooth with no moss on them and I stacked them up on top of this rock. I built a cairn, to mark the death of my previous life. I figured that if moss grew on the rocks it would signal life renewed, and I've been coming up here ever since."

"There's moss growing on them all now, how long ago was that?"

"Seven years ago, to the day."

Her friend smiled, reached out and held her hand. "We were diagnosed the same year," she recalled, "I remember when I joined the Team after I'd finished my chemo, I didn't have the strength to paddle so you suggested I drum."

"Yes, I remember that, you had a good beat."

"It was in tune with my heart back then."

"And now, my friend?"

"I'm not in tune with anything anymore."

"Yes, you are," Ariena contradicted, "you're in tune with nature, you respond to nature's call otherwise you wouldn't perceive the tangible energy all around us." She took her friend's other hand and squeezed it. "You can use nature's energy to bring back your own life force, you just have to want to do it."

"I know, but I don't have the will anymore. I'm tired Ari," she said, "I've just finished my fourth bout of chemo and the cancer hasn't gone. They wont give me anymore, I'm done."

"You're done with chemo, and that's a good thing," Ariena replied, "now maybe your immune system will have a chance to recuperate."

"I have been juicing and eating more fruits and vegetables, but you know me, I love my junk food!"

"Your problem is that you love your junk food more than yourself," Ariena retorted angrily.

"You're right, you're absolutely right, but I don't think I'm worth it."

Ariena turned and hugged her friend. "Don't say that, everyone is worth it, and you especially," she chided.

"There's so much going on at home that isn't working for me, I don't have the support that you do."

"That's all the more reason why you have to love and support yourself. Even with support from family and friends, ultimately we all know that we're alone in this. It's up to each of us to love ourselves enough to make the difference to our outcome," Ariena said, "you have to choose to do it."

Her friend sighed. "I know what you're saying is true, because it's working for you, but it's too late for me, I guess I've made the wrong choices all along."

A gust of cold wind sent a chill through Ariena. "We'd better be going," she said, pulling her friend's hat down to cover her ears, "but you listen to me. There's no right and wrong choices, my friend, all the choices you make will affect your life in one of two ways, either positive or negative. The way I see it, there's only one choice."

Her friend looked at her sadly. "No, Ariena, there are two choices," she said, "you either choose to live, or you don't." Another chill shot through Ariena, but this time there was no wind.

\*

Ariena ran slowly up the trail, watching ahead as she climbed amongst the scattered rocks, the squeak of her footsteps in the snow the only sound. She felt the snow fall and melt on her face as tiny snowflakes drifted by, blown gently on the wind. As she reached the tree line, she stopped and turned to look at the scene below, and smiled sadly at the line of footprints she had left behind. A light dusting of snow had settled on the cedars, their branches hanging low over the trail as she turned to enter the forest. "You never got to leave the first footprints in the snow, did you my friend?" she spoke aloud.

The tree stump was draped in white, the surrounding area sparkled with shards of light where the snow had settled. A little bird flittered amongst the branches, feeding on the tiny red berries still clinging to the bushes below. Ariena stood still, watching the bird as it flew from branch to branch, pecking and dropping berries on the ground. Then she saw it. A perfect paw print etched in the snow, the spirit bear had marked the spot. She knew this was the place to built the cairn.

A tear rolled down her cheek as she placed the last rock on top. She stood back behind the little cairn she had built, and looked out over the trees in the valley below. Far in the distance she could see a tiny black silhouette moving slowly across the water, and as she watched, a gentle breeze wafted up the mountain and brushed her cheek. The miniature boat stopped moving and a faint sound drifted towards her. In tune with her heartbeat, the sound of the drum reverberated through her soul. Her eyes misted over and the image dissolved as she stood still, not wiping the tears as they flowed uncontrollably. She reached into her pocket, pulled out a small brown paper bag and poured the contents into her hand. The sound of the drum faded away and she blinked to clear her eyes. She folded her fingers over the ash in her hand and slowly tipped some onto the cairn.

A tear dropped, and she watched as the tear made a tiny rivulet through the ash. A shrill cry filled the air, and as she looked up, a lone eagle circled once overhead, then was gone. She lifted her arm up above her and opened her hand. Swirling upwards with the breeze, the fine ash drifting slowly away, scattering over the mountain as it fell.

"Fly free, my friend," she whispered, "fly free."

# CHAPTER 14
# SHARING

Ariena and her husband walked slowly towards their car. With his arm around her shoulders, Glen leaned over and kissed her cheek. "Hmm, salty," he said, smiling at her. She wiped the tears away with the back of her hand. "I'm not going to any more funerals," she said, "I'm done with it. How many funerals can you go to in one year? It's not right."

"I know what you mean, it just doesn't seem fair."

"In the past ten years since I was diagnosed, there's more people who have died of cancer than I care to think about, and that's only among people I know!" Ariena said, "Your poor cousin died because she didn't realise that her lifestyle was killing her, and when she did get sick, she didn't know what to do. She was never told what the options are."

"Even when they do know, I don't understand why people make the choices they do," he said shaking his head.

"Tell me about it," Ariena said, thinking back to three years earlier when she stood alone on the mountain, wracked with grief for the loss of her dear friend. "I've spent every day for ten years trying to help people understand how simple it is. My teammates, my friends, our own family, why wont they listen?" She burst into tears and turned into his arms.

"You've helped hundreds of people, sweetheart," he said soothingly, "remember how you were booked solid with consultations when we first opened our Health Centre, and just think of all the people who went on the lifestyle programs you established because you couldn't keep up with all those consultations. They've all made changes that have benefitted their health, not to mention how our restaurant and juice bar showed folks how easy it is to add more raw and vegan food in their diet. Even your parent's health changed dramatically, at their age they were great examples of how the body can rejuvenate," he added. He pushed her hair back and kissed her forehead. "What about the raw food classes and public speaking we've been doing here for the past two years," he continued, "hundreds more people have made conscious lifestyle choices to improve their health because of what they've learnt attending those."

"I know," she said, "but sometimes I feel like we're not reaching enough people. There are more cases of cancer now than there were 10 years ago, and it's because the majority of people don't know that they can take control of their own health. They don't know the truth!"

"I think that there are some who do know, but they just don't think about it," he replied, "the other day I was walking out of the hardware store, and a group of people were cooking up sausages on the barbecue outside, to raise money for cancer research! I couldn't believe it! There they were, using the most carcinogenic form of cooking processed food, to raise money for cancer research!" he shook his head, "Honestly, everyone knows carcinogens cause cancer."

"You see it everywhere," Ariena agreed, "it's like the RSPCA having a hotdog stand to raise awareness for animal cruelty! They just aren't giving it a thought."

"I was reading the sign at the sausage sizzle," he said, "it read 'do you realise that 1 in 2 people will have cancer in their lifetime'. So when they asked if I'd like to buy a sausage, I said no thanks, I'd rather be the 1 in 2 people that don't get cancer, but I don't think they got it."

"You see how frustrating it is," she replied, "there are just so many who don't get it at all! I remember it was 1 in 9 when I was diagnosed, and now, ten years later it's down to 1 in 2. There's something seriously wrong with this picture, we have to do something, people have to be told! Unless we go everywhere spreading the word like the preachers used to do, I don't think we can reach them all." Ariena looked thoughtful. "You know, that's not a bad idea," she said.

"Preaching? I don't think that would go down very well."

"No, I mean going everywhere," she replied, "we've only ever reached our own community, but what if we were to do some kind of tour, you know, travel around speaking."

"I don't know," he said doubtfully, "how many people are going to come and listen, they wont even know who we are or what we've accomplished."

"What if the tour itself was accomplishing something that caught their attention," Ariena was thinking aloud, "what if *we* were to be doing something on the tour that showed by example what can be achieved by living a conscious lifestyle."

"Oh-oh, where are you going with this?" He shot her a knowing look. She smiled at him, her eyes sparkling with excitement. "What if we were to *run* around the country while we do a speaking tour!"

"I knew it," he laughed, as he took her in his arms and kissed her on the nose. "I knew you were still in there. I knew going to that funeral would not hold you down for long," he added, kissing her again, "But *running* around the country? I suppose you'll want to run a marathon every day, just to really prove the point?"

"Yes, of course," she agreed, "a marathon a day should catch their attention! Really though," she said earnestly, "we know it can be done, so why not?"

"Okay," he smiled, "here comes that raw courage that you've shown since the day of your diagnosis, and yes, if it can be done, you're the one to do it."

"*We*," she corrected him, "I seem to recall you saying once that we're in this together, right?"

"Absolutely," he laughed, "but running around the country is going to take a bit of organising so I don't think we can do it this year, there is something you could do this year that would be very appropriate, now that it's been ten years since your diagnosis."

"Oh, really?" she smiled, "you mean celebrate?"

"In a way, yes," he replied, "but this celebration can be shared with thousands of people."

"What do you mean?"

"Well," he said, as he stopped walking and looked at her. "I think it's time you wrote the book. After all, I recall *you* saying that you would share your experience and knowledge in a book after ten years. Well, the time has come, my love. Your story needs to be heard, and as a book, it could reach many people. When they read it, then they'll know the raw truth about how to achieve optimal health, and they can make their own informed choices. At the very least, it will make them think more consciously about the choices they do make in life." Ariena stood very still for a moment, then slowly she looked up at him. "You're right," she said, "it is time."

"That's my girl," he said, bending down and kissing her full on the mouth. She melted in his arms, returning his kiss with the same passion they had shared for over forty years. "Let's go home," he murmured in her ear, "no more funerals, there's too much living to do." Ariena felt a sudden wave of excitement as she turned to the man she loved.

"Yes, life is for *living*, everyone needs to know how simple and easy and joyful it can be." She put her hand in his and squeezed it. "And life is for loving," she added.

"What will you call it?" he asked, smiling at her. She thought for a moment, then a knowing look brightened her face. "I think it should be called Raw Can Cure anything, including CANCER."

"That's it," he agreed, "end of story!"

*

Chapter 14   *Sharing*

# Chapter 14    *Sharing*

# RUNNING OUT OF TIME

*An extract from Janette Murray-Wakelin's new book.*

"Throughout the year 2013, as veteran raw vegan runners, my husband Alan and I ran together around Australia: 15,782 kilometres, averaging 43 kilometers, a marathon everyday. Step for step, stride for stride all the way. We started in Melbourne, Victoria on January 1, 2013, following Highway 1 around the perimeter of the country running through every State Capital and finished running 365 marathons in 365 days back in Melbourne December 31, 2013. On January 1, 2014, we ran one more marathon (number 366) from Melbourne to Warrandyte along the Yarra River Trail, thereby setting a new World Record for running the most consecutive marathons as the oldest and only couple to run around Australia, fueled entirely by fruit and vegetables and wearing barefoot shoes.

We wanted to inspire and motivate others to make more conscious lifestyle choices, to promote kindness and compassion for all living beings and to raise environmental awareness for a sustainable future. The truth is, the most endangered species on this planet is Humankind. As a species, we have become obsessed with speed, the Human Race is on, but we are not winning. Through misinformation and misleading marketing, we are disregarding the innate intelligence of our own bodies and have become a malnourished species, while the sickness industry flourishes. Due to our poor food choices we have become a species of (non) survivors. The majority of us are spending most of our lives dying instead of thriving. The amount of money and time spent on 'scientific research' to find a cure for our ill health would be better spent on prevention and returning to our natural way of being. Our obsession with technology has us careering down a path of self destruction. In our rush to become technically advanced we have lost sight of the importance of Being. Our poor lifestyle choices are creating our own demise, we are spiraling into oblivion, and we are Running Out of Time.

We believe that the Human Race needs to slow down and heed what one of our greatest teachers, Gandhi in his wisdom told us, "There is more to life than increasing it's speed." We need to revisit who we are and why we are here. We need to understand the consequences of the choices we make in life and how they can affect our very being.

By doing so, we *can* make a difference. Awareness comes through being informed with truth, understanding the information and acting on it, but knowledge requires action to become conscious awareness.

We wanted to share a positive message of truth and hope from the experiences and knowledge that we had gained through living consciously during the previous decade, so that others may make their own informed lifestyle choices that *will* make a difference. We knew the best way to do that was to lead by example, walk (or in this case) run the talk. Inspiration is what motivates people to never stop pushing for what they believe in and for what they want to achieve. By running a marathon distance together every day for a year around Australia, we hoped to inspire others to think more consciously about the choices they make in life, to believe in themselves, to follow their dreams, and to achieve their goals. While we were Running around Australia during the year 2013, we had the opportunity to show that by eating raw living plant based foods, we are healthier, more physically fit and have unlimited energy at beyond 60 years of age than in our earlier years, including when we ran the length of New Zealand 13 years previously.

We have been enjoying unlimited energy for over 12 years due primarily to our 100% Low Fat Raw Vegan Diet. A vegan diet is based on fresh, ripe, organic fruits and vegetables with NO animal products. A 100 percent low fat, raw, vegan diet is based on the 80/10/10 principle of 80 percent carbohydrates, 10 percent protein and 10 percent fat derived from fresh, ripe, organic fruits and vegetables. A low fat, raw vegan 80/10/10 diet does NOT include any animal products, processed or junk foods and does NOT include any stimulants, drugs, supplements nor 'superfoods'. By eliminating all acid-forming foods (everything *other* than fresh ripe fruits and vegetables) and increasing the amount of alkaline foods in our diet, (obtained *only* from fresh, ripe fruits and vegetables) we have attained a higher level of optimum health, improved our physical fitness and increased our performance level.

In our experience, unlimited Raw Energy is attained by consuming an abundance of high nutrient- laden, fresh, ripe, organic fruits and vegetables. It is also our experience that true happiness is attained through making conscious lifestyle choices for one's own health, the health of the environment, and all living beings with whom we share the planet. We are living proof of what can be achieved by making conscious lifestyle choices.

So many times we've been asked, "Where do you get your protein?" The answer is simple: "The same place that the cow gets it from - greens." Protein from plant based sources is healthier than the protein derived from animal sources and does not contribute to health issues such as heart dis-ease and cancer. It is much more efficient for people to consume the plant food directly. We are also asked where we get our calcium, or iron, or any other nutrients a person thinks to name. Again, the answer is that we get all our necessary nutrients from the food we eat, just the same as animals in their natural habitat do. Malnutrition is unknown in people and animals who eat raw living food in abundance. We live in a world where over 790 million people are chronically undernourished and over 27,000 children under the age of five die of malnutrition every day. The world's cattle consume enough plant food to feed 8.7 billion people, more than the entire human population. Available protein from plants that the animals eat and 80-95 percent of food energy is wasted when converted to meat for human consumption. Cooking food also reduces the available nutrients and enzymes essential for optimum health. By nourishing our bodies with raw living vegan foods, humans not only can achieve optimal physical, mental and spiritual health, but can also acquire unlimited Raw Energy which enables us to achieve our goals and follow our dreams. Raw Energy is already achieved by every other free animal on the planet. The good news is that Raw Energy is readily available to humans just by making informed conscious lifestyle choices. Living a conscious lifestyle is a safe, sure way to get back on track with your health and ensures optimal health and happiness, the two things that everyone is ultimately striving for. Everyone can benefit from learning how to take control of their own health and therefore feel good about themselves. It is immensely gratifying to see how even small changes can make such a difference in one's life and having the right information empowers one to make conscious life choices. All dis-ease and related health issues are reversible through maintaining all aspects of a conscious living lifestyle. Becoming conscious of the lifestyle choices we make personally and collectively as a community and a species, will help to bring about the change to a more sustainable future for ourselves, our children and future generations."

'Running Out of Time,' is based on the author's experiences while running around Australia during 2013. It includes her daily writings on each marathon, images from the Run and 'Recipes from the Road,' a precursor to her upcoming raw vegan recipe book.

**www.RawVeganPath.com**

# READER'S REVIEWS

*"I have just finished reading your book - Raw Can Cure Cancer. Thank you so much for this inspiring book!"* - Daniela, Switzerland

*"Thank you for your insightful and healthful information"* - Maurice , USA

*"I am very inspired by your story, well done you are a true inspiration"* - Emma , Australia

*"Your book made be laugh, it made me cry and it made me think, thank you"* - Narelle , Australia

*"Just read your book, awesome!"* - Trina , Australia

*"A wonderful mix of interesting and inspiring"* - Sam , Singapore

*"My wife and I find your story inspirational"* - Brian , USA

*"Just finished reading your book, thank you for sharing the message"* - Jo , Australia

*"Thank you for sharing your wisdom"* - Kay , Australia

*"Thank you for sharing your inspirational story. I will cure my body and health through your inspiration"* - Bob , USA

*"I have just read your book and love it! Thanks for your work"* - Kathy , Australia

*"I love your story, thank you for sharing"* - Danielle , Australia

*"I have just finished your book about your cancer journey. I am inspired by your courage and thrilled to have such a great book to recommend to friends. You are doing a truly wonderful thing, thank you"* - Mary, Australia

*"I am so inspired by your story, you gave me hope"* - Felicia , Australia

*"Just reading your book, it totally resonates with me, well done on getting this info out there"* - Pauline, Singapore

*"You have given me hope, what a blessing you are"* - Melanie, UK

*"What a blessing to read your inspiring story"* - Laurie, UK

*"I loved your book, so much information and so well written. It's very inspirational"* - Diana, Australia

*"Your book needs to be in every home, it should be mandatory reading in schools"* - Jon, Australia

*"Everyone should read this book, so inspirational"* - Penny, Australia

*"I love the way this book is written, so easy to resonate with so many messages"* - Guy, USA

*"Finally...a book on cancer that tells the truth"* - William

*"This book really draws the reader into the story, very well written and so informative"* - Jen

# Raw

## CAN CURE CANCER

ISBN 9781922175779                                                      Qty

RRP        AU$26.99        .....

Postage within Australia        AU$5.00        .....

TOTAL★  $_____

★ All prices include GST

Name:................................................................................................................

Address: ...........................................................................................................

..........................................................................................................................

Phone:..............................................................................................................

Email: ...............................................................................................................

Payment: ❏ Money Order ❏ Cheque ❏ MasterCard ❏Visa

Cardholder's Name:........................................................................................

Credit Card Number: .....................................................................................

Signature:.........................................................................................................

Expiry Date: ....................................................................................................

Allow 7 days for delivery.

Payment to:        Marzocco Consultancy (ABN 14 067 257 390)
PO Box 12544
A'Beckett Street, Melbourne, 8006 VIC, Australia
admin@brolgapublishing.com.au

BE PUBLISHED

Publish through a successful publisher.
Brolga Publishing is represented through:
• **National** book trade distribution, including sales,
  marketing & distribution through **Macmillan Australia.**
• **International** book trade distribution to
  • The United Kingdom
  • North America
  • Sales representation in South East Asia
• **Worldwide e-Book distribution**

For details and inquiries, contact:
Brolga Publishing Pty Ltd
PO Box 12544
A'Beckett St VIC 8006

Phone: 0414 608 494
admin@brolgapublishing.com.au
markzocchi@brolgapublishing.com.au
ABN: 46 063 962 443
(Email for a catalogue request)

CPSIA information can be obtained
at www.ICGtesting.com
Printed in the USA
LVHW011400090721
692305LV00014B/1105